Atlas of Psoriatic Arthritis

P.J. Mease and P.S. Helliwell (Eds.)

Atlas of
Psoriatic Arthritis

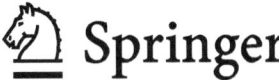 Springer

P.J. Mease, MED (RHUUH)
University of Washington
  School of Medicine
Seattle, WA
USA

P.S. Helliwell, DM, PhD, FRCP
Academic Unit of Musculoskeletal and
  Rehabilitation Medicine
University of Leeds
Leeds, UK

British Library Cataloguing in Publication Data

Atlas of psoriatic arthritis
  1. Psoriatic arthritis—Atlases
  I. Mease, P. J.   II. Helliwell, Philip, 1947–
  616.5′26

  ISBN-13: 9781846288968

Library of Congress Control Number: 2007928819

ISBN: 978-1-84628-896-8 (HB)   e-ISBN: 978-1-84628-897-5
ISBN: 978-0-85729-174-5 (PB)

9 8 7 6 5 4 3 2 1

Springer Science+Business Media
springer.com

Contents

Contributors

Jennifer Barton
University of California
San Francisco Medical Center
San Francisco, CA, USA

Kristina P. Callis
Utah Psoriasis Initiative
University of Utah
Salt Lake City, UT, USA

Helen Foster
School of Clinical Medical Sciences
Newcastle University
Newcastle, UK

Dafna D. Gladman
University of Toronto
  School of Medicine
Toronto, Ontario, Canada

P. S. Helliwell
Academic Unit of Musculoskeletal and
  Rehabilitation Medicine
University of Leeds
Leeds, UK

Gerald G. Krueger
Utah Psoriasis Initiative
University of Utah
Salt Lake City, UT, USA

Dennis McGonagle
Academic Unit of Musculoskeletal Disease
University of Leeds
Leeds, UK

P. J. Mease
University of Washington School
  of Medicine
Seattle, WA, USA

Christopher Ritchlin
University of Rochester
School of Medicine and Dentistry
Rochester, NY, USA

Ai Lyn Tan
Academic Unit of Musculoskeletal Disease
University of Leeds
Leeds, UK

Introduction

P. J. Mease and P. S. Helliwell

Although initially thought to be a variant of rheumatoid arthritis (RA), the pioneering work of Wright and Baker identified the distinctive features of the arthritis occurring in association with psoriasis [1]. Wright described the frequent involvement of the distal Interphalangeal (DIP) joints with erosion and absorption of the terminal phalanges and frequent reduction of bone stock in the other digits leading to a mutilating form of arthritis. Wright also described sacroiliitis and spondylitis occurring alone and in association with peripheral arthritis. The original five clinical sub-groups described by Moll and Wright are still in use today although the validity of this classification has been challenged [2] (*see* Figure 3.1).

Wright and Moll later defined the concept of the seronegative spondyloarthropathies as a group of disorders sharing common clinical features including (as a hallmark feature) sacroiliitis, a seronegative (for rheumatoid factor) anodular asymmetrical peripheral oligoarthritis, a hyperkeratotic and sometimes pustular rash on the hands and soles (keratoderma blenorrhagica), peripheral and central enthesitis, anterior uveitis, and familial aggregation [3]. The discovery of the high prevalence of HLA-B27 in ankylosing spondylitis and other diseases in this group provided confirmation of this concept. Psoriatic arthritis (PsA) fit very well into the spondyloarthropathy group, often demonstrating many of the shared clinical features described above. It is, therefore, sometimes difficult to differentiate PsA from other spondyloarthropathies such as reactive arthritis and ankylosing spondylitis (*see* Figure 3.5).

Despite clinical, radiological and familial evidence supporting PsA as a distinct disease entity, controversy still exists about which patient to include within this disease group. Some authors have even questioned whether PsA is a separate disease, suggesting that psoriasis merely modifies the expression of pre-existing RA. Other authors have argued that new onset chronic polyarthritis is undifferentiated and only evolves into a more distinctive form with time such that the presence of psoriasis at onset of disease is of no value in nosological terms [4]. The problem is not with the classical presentation of PsA – with oligoarthritis, DIP involvement, calcaneal enthesitis, and dactylitis – but with the group of patients who have seronegative polyarthritis and psoriasis.

Overall, the sex ratio in PsA approximates unity but will vary across the sub-groups so that male predominance occurs in the spondylitis and oligoarthritis groups while females predominate in the most frequent sub-group, symmetrical polyarthritis, as also occurs in RA.

The peak age of onset of PsA is similar to that found in RA (20–40 years). This is, in most cases, later than the onset of psoriasis so that psoriasis precedes arthritis in the majority of cases. However, a potential source of diagnostic confusion occurs when arthritis precedes psoriasis, as it does in 15–20% of cases [5]. For this reason, it is important for the physician to check thoroughly for clinical stigmata of psoriasis including examination of the nails, scalp, the soles and palms, and the flexural areas, particularly the natal cleft (*see* Figure 3.18).

Clinical evaluation of patients with suspected PsA should, therefore, be systematic and include an assessment of the skin, the entheses and the spine. The importance of family history cannot be overemphasised because of the familial clustering initially described by Wright and others. Evaluation of the established case should include an assessment of the skin and joints taking into account the distinctive features of PsA. Although there are well established ways of measuring the skin involvement, many people make a quasi-objective appraisal and record 'mild, moderate or severe'. From the articular point of view, evaluation involves performing a 68 tender joint/66 swollen joint count to include the DIP joints, assessing the presence of dactylitis and enthesitis, and the severity of spinal involvement, if relevant. In the clinic situation it often helps to have a proforma to aid this complex assessment process and to facilitate recording of data. Radiological studies can help clarify the diagnosis with a minimum plain radiographic set of hands, feet, and pelvis as the frequency of asymptomatic sacroiliitis in PsA should alert the physician to X-ray these joints if there is diagnostic suspicion of this disease. In early disease, when plain radiographs are normal, magnetic resonance imaging (MRI) can be of help as MRI changes precede plain radiographic abnormalities (*see* Chapter 4, *Imaging*).

References

1. Wright V. **Psoriatic arthritis: a comparative study of rheumatoid arthritis and arthritis associated with psoriasis.** *Ann Rheum Dis* 1961;**20**:123.
2. Helliwell P, Marchesoni A, Peters M *et al*. **A re-evaluation of the osteoarticular manifestations of psoriasis.** *Br J Rheumatol* 1991;**30**:339–345.
3. Wright V, Moll JMH. *Seronegative Polyarthritis.* Amsterdam: North Holland Publishing Co., 1976.
4. Harrison BJ, Silman AJ, Barrell EM *et al*. **Presence of psoriasis does not influence the presentation or short-term outcome of patients with early inflammatory polyarthritis.** *J Rheumatol* 1997;**24**:1744–1749.
5. Gladman DD, Shuckelt R, Russell ML *et al*. **Psoriatic arthritis (PSA) – an analysis of 220 patients.** *Q J Med* 1987;**238**:127–141.

1
Epidemiology

Dafna D. Gladman

Psoriatic arthritis (PsA) has been defined as an inflammatory arthritis, usually seronegative for rheumatoid factor, associated with psoriasis [1]. Other clinical features associated with PsA include the presence of spondylitis and sacroiliitis, dactylitis (swelling of the whole digit), enthesitis (inflammation at tendon insertion), and extra-articular manifestations of seronegative spondyloarthropathies such as iritis, urethritis, inflammatory bowel changes, and aortic root dilatation. The original description of PsA was that of a mild disease compared with rheumatoid arthritis (RA) [2]. Moll and Wright described five clinical patterns of PsA:

- predominantly distal joint disease, with distal interphalangeal (DIP) joint involvement;
- an oligoarthritis, usually asymmetric;
- a symmetric polyarthritis indistinguishable from RA;
- arthritis mutilans; and
- spondyloarthritis.

Subsequent authors have had difficulty recognizing all the patterns and suggested other methods for the classification of PsA [3]. Several proposed methods of classification have been published, but none has been widely accepted or validated. A current examination of the classification of PsA suggests that most of these methods function well in distinguishing patients with PsA from patients with other inflammatory arthritis; however, a new classification was developed by the CASPAR (ClASsification of Psoriatic ARthritis) group [4].

Patients with PsA have a reduced quality of life compared with the general population and various instruments have been developed to measure this. Patients with PsA suffer from fatigue more frequently than the general population. This was demonstrated by the administration of a modification of the Krupp Fatigue Severity Score (FSS) [5,6]. This nine-item scale assesses the impact of fatigue on activities of daily living and is scored from 0 to 10, with higher scores indicating more severe fatigue. The FSS for 75 patients with PsA was higher than for the 100 healthy controls (5.2 ± 3.0 versus 3.9 ± 2.1, $p = 0.001$). A total of 45% of the PsA patients reported the presence of fatigue on clinical assessment. The mean FSS score in this group was 6.9 compared with 3.8 in patients who did not report fatigue. Fatigue was associated with fibromyalgia, tender joint count, morning stiffness, clinically damaged joint count, actively inflamed joint count, and hemoglobin [6]. Change in FSS over time, analyzed for 90 patients with PsA, was found to be related to changes in actively inflamed joints, suggesting that fatigue reflects joint disease activity in these patients [7]. Recently, the Functional Assessment of Chronic Illness Therapy (FACIT) Fatigue Scale was validated in PsA. The FACIT-Fatigue was reproducible and correlated with other fatigue measures as well as with disease activity in patients with PsA [8]. It was shown to be responsive to treatment in the ADEPT (Abnormal Doppler Enteral Prescription Trial) study [9].

Genetic factors are thought to contribute significantly to the susceptibility and expression of both psoriasis and PsA, and some overlap between the genetic susceptibilities to the two diseases is likely. Therefore, informative data can be gathered by following the transmission of psoriasis along with PsA when attempting to elucidate the genetic basis of PsA. Evidence for the importance of genetic factors comes from family investigations, human leukocyte antigen studies, and genome scans; the latter being performed primarily in psoriasis.

Some 40% of patients with PsA have a family history of either psoriasis or PsA in a first-degree relative. Twin studies in psoriasis reveal that monozygotic twins are concordant for psoriasis much more than dizygotic twins. A total of 40% of the patients in our longitudinal cohort provided a family history of either psoriasis or PsA. Of the PsA patients, 48% reported a parent with psoriasis or PsA that may not have been previously recognized [10]. Twin studies in psoriasis reveal a concordance rate for monozygotic twins of 62–70% compared with 21–23% for dizygotic twins [11–13]. A very recent twin study from Denmark failed to identify an increased prevalence of PsA with one of 10 monozygotic twins and two of 25 dizygotic twins. However, the study was based on a small sample of 35 twin pairs [14]. A segregation study in psoriasis concluded that a polygenic or multifactorial pattern is the most likely mode of inheritance [15]. There are no reports of segregation studies in PsA. A family investigation of 100 patients with PsA and 20 patients with psoriasis who did not have arthritis demonstrated that 12.5% of the PsA patients had relatives with documented PsA, whereas none of the relatives of patients with psoriasis had relatives with PsA [16]. Applying Risch's analysis [17] the relative risk for a first-degree relative (λ_1) is 55, and the risk for siblings (λ_s) is 27.

Clearly, further studies are required to identify the genetic predisposition to PsA both among patients with psoriasis and among the general population. These will require large numbers of patients and families from diverse ethnic backgrounds, and are likely to depend on international collaboration. Studies relating genetic factors to disease expression in PsA are currently ongoing.

Typical psoriatic lesions in a patient with PsA

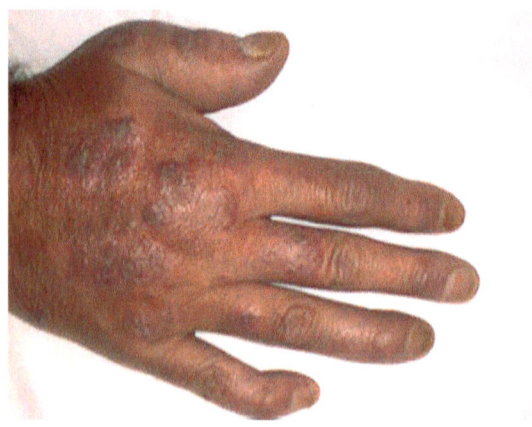

FIGURE 1.1. Plaques are sharply demarcated, erythematous, and have a silvery-white surface scale. This patient also exhibits some of the nail changes that are common in psoriasis, namely dystrophy, pitting and accumulation of subungual debris. There is no direct relation between the severity of skin lesions and the degree of joint inflammation in psoriatic arthritis (PsA).

Incidence and prevalence data for PsA in published studies

Author	Site	Source	Incidence /100,000	Prevalence /100,000
O'Neill & Silman [18]	Faroe Islands	Population-based	NA	1500
Kaipiainen-Seppanen [19]	Finland	Medication database	6.8	NA
Shbeeb et al. [20]	Rochester, USA	Population-based	6.59	100
Hukuda et al. [21]	Japan	Referrals to medical centers	0.06	1.2
Soderlin et al. [22]	Southern Sweden	Population-based referral study	8	NA
Savolainen et al. [23]	Kuopio, Finland	Referrals for inflammatory arthritis related to total population	23.2	NA
Alamanos et al. [24]	Northwest Greece	Population survey	3.02	56.5
Minaur et al. [25]	Queensland, Australia	Aboriginal survey	NA	1500

FIGURE 1.2. Exact incidence and prevalence rates of PsA are not known. Incidence estimates vary from 3 to 23 per 100,000 individuals in a given population, whereas prevalence estimates range from 1.2 to 1500 per 100,000 in published studies. Partly due to the lack of valid and widely accepted classification criteria, and partly due to the fact that it may be difficult to diagnose PsA at the bedside [26], it is likely that the rates published to date underestimate the true figures for incidence and prevalence. NA, not available.

Prevalence of PsA among patients with psoriasis

Author	Year	Center	No. psoriasis patients	% patients with PsA
Leczinsky [27]	1948	Sweden	534	7
Vilanova & Pinol [28]	1951	Barcelona	214	25
Little *et al.* [29]	1975	Toronto	100	32
Scarpa *et al.* [30]	1984	Napoli	180	34
Stern [31]	1985	Boston	1285	20
Zanelli & Wilde [32]	1992	Winston-Salem	459	17
Barišic-Druško *et al.* [33]	1994	Osijek region	553	10
Salvarani *et al.* [34]	1995	Regio Emilia	205	36
Shbeeb *et al.* [35]	2000	Mayo Clinic	1056	6.25
Brockbank *et al.* [36]	2001	Toronto	126	31
Alenius *et al.* [37]	2002	Sweden	276	48
National Psoriasis Foundation	2002	USA	4.4 million	23
Zachariae [38]	2003	Denmark	5795	30

FIGURE 1.3. Several investigators have attempted to identify the prevalence of PsA among patients with psoriasis. These figures have varied from 6% to 48%. As noted above, because there are no widely accepted criteria for the diagnosis or classification of PsA, the prevalence of the disease may be underestimated, even among patients with psoriasis. Most recent figures suggest a frequency of 30%, which is probably accurate.

Predominantly DIP joint involvement in PsA

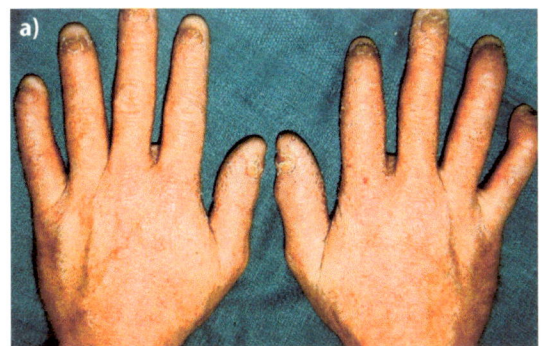
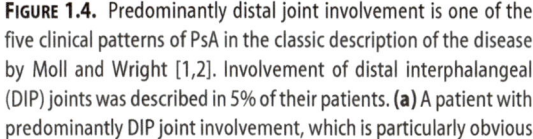
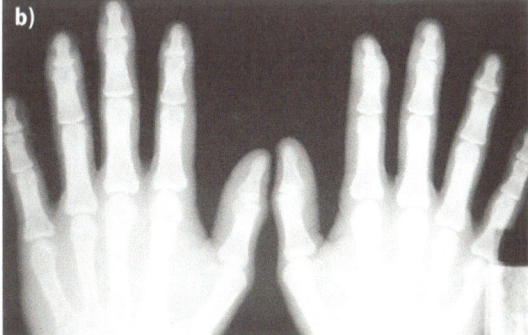

FIGURE 1.4. Predominantly distal joint involvement is one of the five clinical patterns of PsA in the classic description of the disease by Moll and Wright [1,2]. Involvement of distal interphalangeal (DIP) joints was described in 5% of their patients. **(a)** A patient with predominantly DIP joint involvement, which is particularly obvious in the right hand. **(b)** Radiograph of the hands of the same patient confirms that DIP joints are affected. Subsequent studies have questioned the presence of these five patterns in PsA. In particular, several investigators have not identified isolated distal joint disease among their patients with PsA [39–41].

Oligoarthritis in patients with PsA

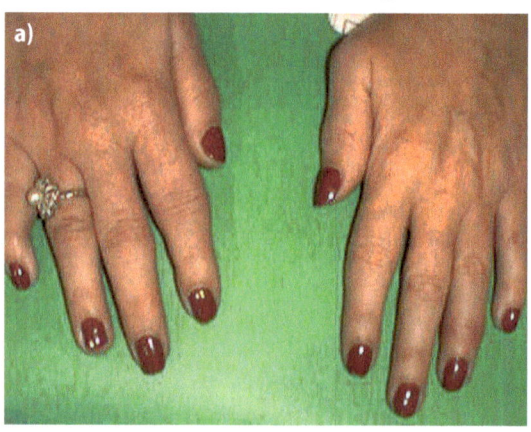 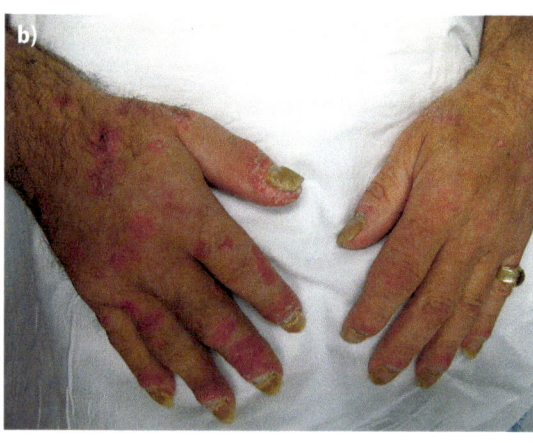

FIGURE 1.5. Oligoarthritis, where fewer than five joints are involved, most often in an asymmetric pattern, was found in the majority of patients (70%) in the Moll and Wright series [2].

(a) Oligoarthritis involving proximal interphalangeal (PIP) joints in both hands. **(b)** A severe case of oligoarthritis affecting mainly the right hand.

Symmetric polyarthritis in PsA

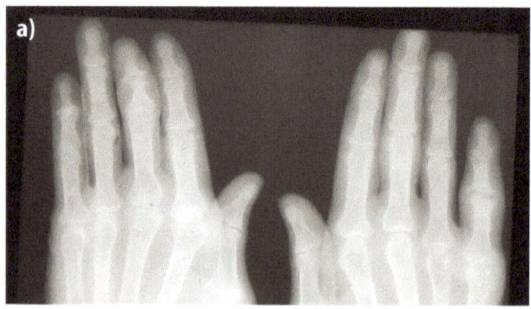 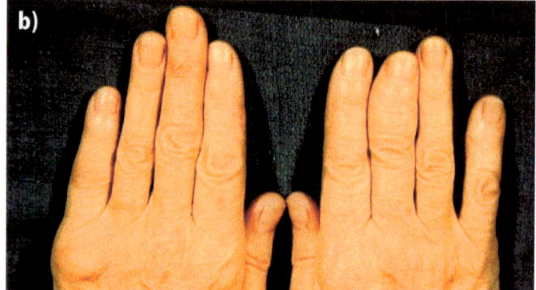

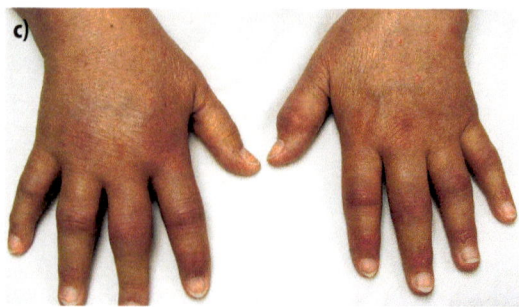

FIGURE 1.6. Symmetric polyarthritis, which is clinically indistinguishable from rheumatoid arthritis (RA), was found in 20% of the patients in the Moll and Wright series [2]. Several studies have demonstrated subsequently that polyarthritis is more common among patients with PsA than initially described [42,43]. **(a,b)** Symmetric polyarthritis in a different patient. There is noticeable involvement of the first PIP joints. **(c)** Symmetric polyarthritis affecting mainly PIP joints.

Arthritis mutilans in PsA

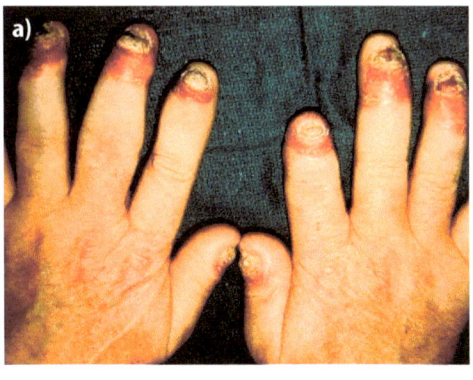
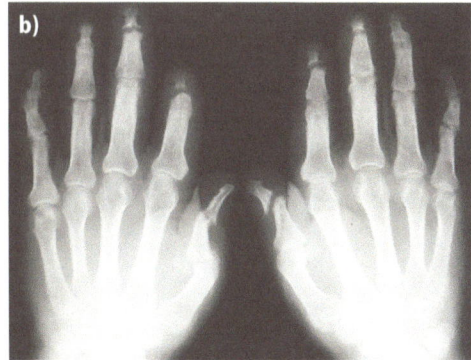

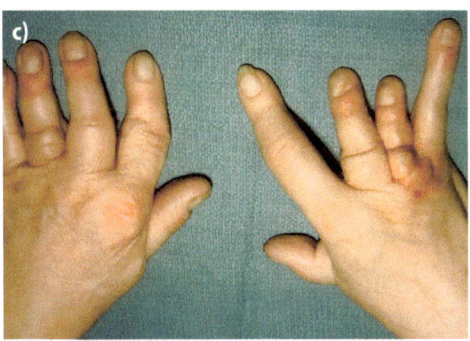
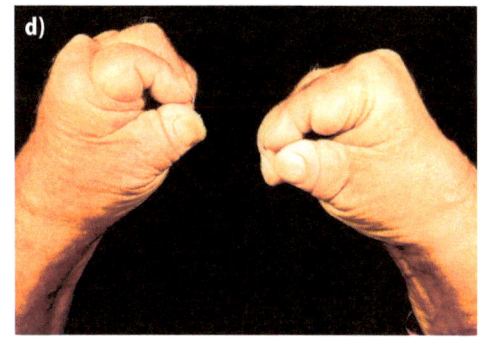

FIGURE 1.7. Arthritis mutilans is a severely destructive form of arthritis. **(a,b)** Polyarthritis, marked psoriatic nail changes, and shortening of the first digit on the right hand are evident in this patient with arthritis mutilans. **(c)** Arthritis mutilans in PsA involving all digits. Some digits are shortened, others show evidence of ankylosis. **(d)** Severe arthritis mutilans in PsA resulting in extreme shortening of all digits.

Spondyloarthritis in PsA

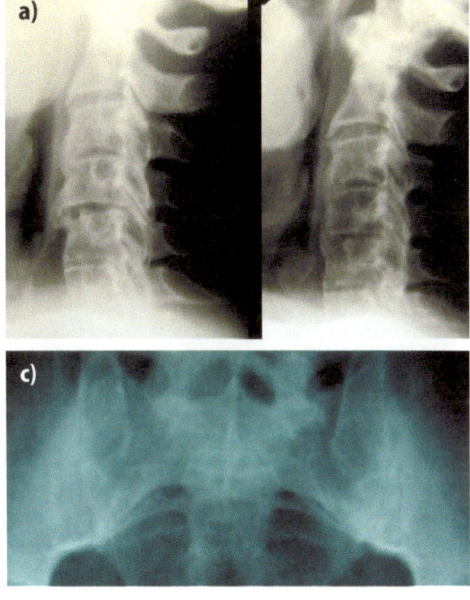
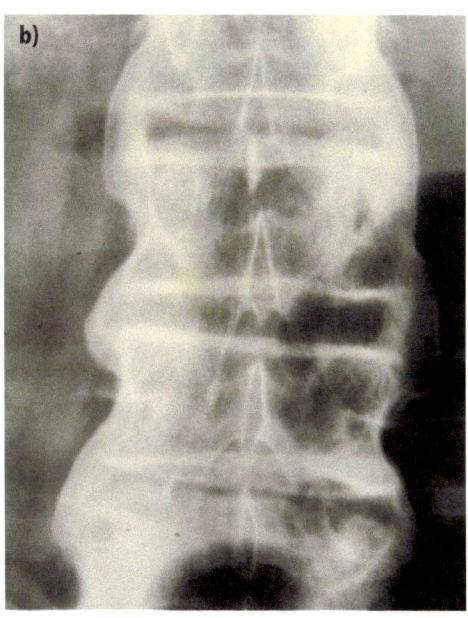

FIGURE 1.8. Syndesmophytes are visible. Isolated spondylitis is rare in PsA. It has been difficult to classify patients who have spondylitis together with peripheral arthritis based on the Moll and Wright classification. Gladman [42] has therefore reformatted the Moll and Wright classifications to include seven categories that are mutually exclusive: distal arthritis, oligoarthritis, polyarthritis, back only, back with distal, back with oligoarthritis, and back with polyarthritis. Arthritis mutilans was not considered a separate class since any of the patterns (except for isolated back involvement) may have features of arthritis mutilans.

Change in patterns of PsA in 664 patients in an inception cohort

First clinic visit	At diagnosis								TOTAL
Arthritis pattern	0	1	2	3	4	5	6	7	First clinic visit
0	**0**	0	2	2	0	1	0	0	**5**
1	0	**22**	6	7	0	0	1	0	**36**
2	0	10	**74**	17	1	1	4	4	**111**
3	0	38	69	**143**	0	3	3	11	**267**
4	0	0	1	4	**15**	0	0	1	**21**
5	0	9	4	2	3	**0**	2	0	**20**
6	0	2	14	3	5	3	**8**	1	**36**
7	0	4	48	54	5	5	11	**41**	**168**
TOTAL at diagnosis	**0**	**85**	**218**	**232**	**29**	**13**	**29**	**58**	**664**

0, remission; 1, distal only; 2, oligoarthritis; 3, polyarthritis; 4, back only; 5, back + distal; 6, back + oligoarthritis; 7, back + polyarthritis

FIGURE 1.9. One of the difficulties in identifying PsA patterns at onset is that patients are not often seen exactly at disease onset and patterns do change over time. This figure depicts the pattern of arthritis recognized by the patient at onset, compared with the pattern observed at the first visit by the physician. Helliwell *et al.* [44] reevaluated the Moll and Wright classification and suggested that three patterns describe patients with PsA: a peripheral arthritis, axial arthritis, and extraosseous manifestations including the SAPHO (synovitis, acne, pustulosis, hyperostosis, and osteitis) syndrome. Veale *et al.* [45] also suggest that there may be an alternate way to describe the patterns seen in PsA. They too suggest three patterns: asymmetric oligoarthritis, symmetric polyarthritis, and spondyloarthritis. Without specific definitions a reduction in the number of patterns may not be more helpful in the classification of PsA. While at presentation the patterns appear to hold true, over time there are changes in pattern. Patients who present with oligoarthritis may accrue more joints and become polyarticular, whereas others who are treated may change from polyarticular to oligoarticular [46,47]. Back involvement occurs later in the course of the disease and requires radiographic evaluation as many patients with PsA and back disease are asymptomatic [48,49]. This leads to difficulties in using clinical patterns for the classification of the disease at its later stages.

Dactylitis in fingers and toes in PsA

a)
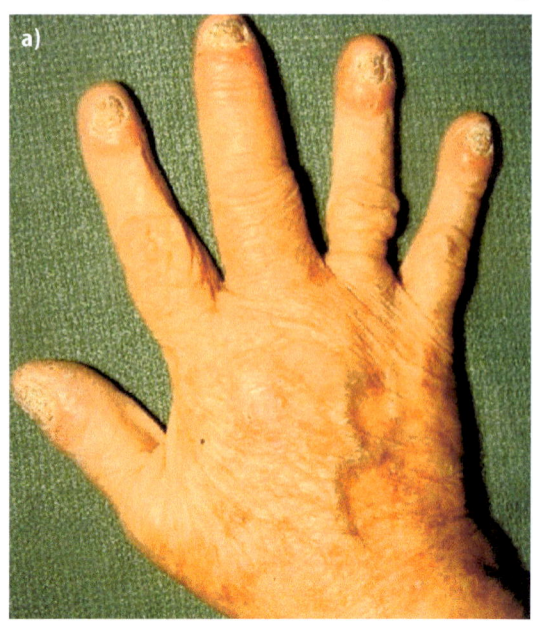

b)
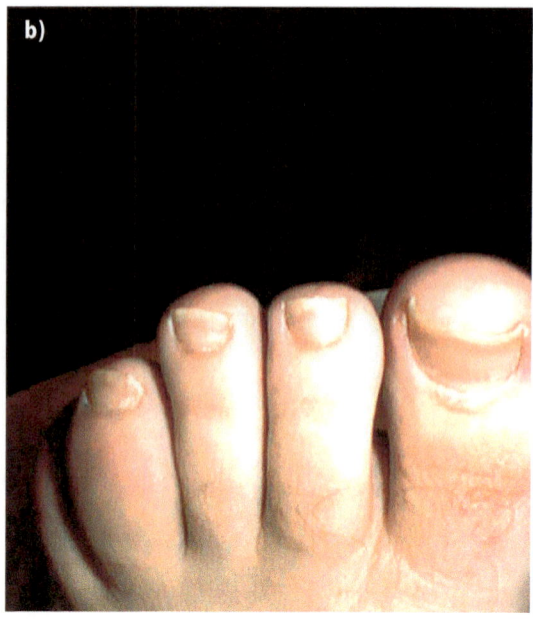

FIGURE 1.10. Some patients may present with dactylitis, in which case the diagnosis is facilitated. Dactylitis is characterized by diffuse swelling of the entire digit, along with arthritis of the joint. It can affect the toes as well as the fingers.

Photograph and radiograph of enthesitis in PsA

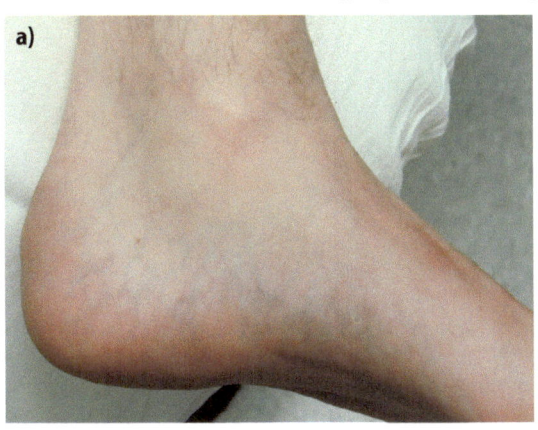

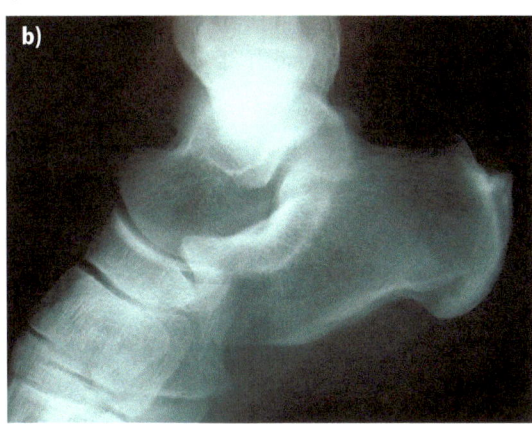

FIGURE 1.11. Patients may present with enthesitis, inflammation of the point of attachment of a tendon, ligament, or joint capsule to a bone. Inflammation commonly leads to formation of new bone at the enthesis. Some investigators have questioned the possibility that enthesitis alone can be a pattern in PsA.

Adjusted mean SF-36 health survey scores for PsA sample and UK and USA general populations

SF-36 scales	PsA	UK	USA	p value*
Physical functioning	68.8	86.2	85.2	0.0001
Social functioning	81.4	88.4	84.6	0.01[†]
Role physical	65.8	84.6	82.9	0.0001
Role emotional	71.4	84.4	82.9	0.05
Mental health	73.0	75.1	75.6	NS
Vitality	57.5	61.7	62.4	NS
Pain	61.5	80.9	74.0	0.0001
General health	58.8	72.0	72.1	0.0001

*p value comparing PsA to UK and USA populations
[†]p value comparing PsA to UK population only

FIGURE 1.12. The Medical Outcome Survey (MOS) Short Form 36 (SF-36) is a generic questionnaire that is commonly used to assess quality of life among patients with rheumatologic disorders [50]. Its advantage is that it allows comparison among patients with different medical conditions. Husted *et al.* studied 113 patients with PsA [51]. They found that the quality of life was lower in patients with PsA compared with both US and UK control groups. The same group also found that the SF-36 was more responsive to changes in clinical status than the Health Assessment Questionnaire (HAQ) or the Arthritis Impact Measurement Scale (AIMS) [52]. A recently developed instrument for assessment of quality of life among patients with PsA also demonstrated reduced quality of life [53]. This instrument was developed through questioning patients with PsA and was validated against other quality-of-life instruments such as the European Quality of Life (EUROQoL) scale. It remains to be seen how it compares with the SF-36 and HAQ, and whether it is responsive to clinical changes. The HAQ was developed specifically for patients with arthritis. It has also been studied in patients with PsA. Patients with PsA demonstrate impaired function compared with healthy controls, as well as compared with patients with RA [54,55]. The HAQ has shown responsiveness in clinical trials in PsA [56,57]. These trials have demonstrated a significant response with an average reduction of 0.6. A minimally clinically important change of 0.3 has been recommended [58]. NS, not significant. Adapted from [51].

Predictive factors for mortality in PsA

Factor	Relative risk	Confidence interval	p value
Prior medication	1.83	0.93, 3.60	0.079
Radiographic damage	3.88	1.32, 11.35	0.014
ESR >15	3.77	1.31, 10.83	0.013
Nail changes	0.33	0.14, 0.76	0.009

FIGURE 1.13. Initially, PsA was thought to be a mild disease but recently it has been demonstrated to be a progressive deforming disease with increased mortality risk. One study suggested that there was good outcome in patients who had been admitted to hospital [59]. However, several recent studies have shown that there is progressive disease over a period of 5 years [60,61]. Studies further document that polyarthritis at presentation is a predictor for pro-gression, as are some genetic markers [62–64]. Indeed, within the first 2 years of PsA 47% of patients had evidence of erosive disease [65]. Patients with PsA have also been shown to have an increased mortality risk compared with the general population [66]. The major causes of death are similar to those of the general population, and previous active and severe disease are predictors for mortality [67]. ESR, erythrocyte sedimentation rate. Adapted from [67].

Factors associated with remission in PsA

Characteristic	Remission group (n=69)	Non-remission group (n=178)	p value
Mean age	42.6	42.0	0.73
Male	49 (71%)	90 (51%)	0.01
Age at onset			
Psoriasis	29.2	28.6	0.77
Arthritis	35.8	34.5	0.44
Disease duration			
Psoriasis	12.7	13.4	0.66
Arthritis	6.1	7.5	0.21
Arthritis pattern			
Peripheral only	45 (73%)	111 (64%)	0.21
Spine	17 (27%)	63 (36%)	
Active joints	6.0	12.8	0.01
Effusions	2.1	3.3	0.01
Deformed joints	2.8	3.3	0.05
Damaged joints	3.2	5.8	0.01
ACR FCI	27 (39%)	39 (22%)	0.01
Neck pain	15 (22%)	65 (37%)	0.02
PASI	8.3	5.4	0.16
No medications	40 (58%)	76 (43%)	0.03
IA injections	15 (22%)	73 (41%)	0.01

FIGURE 1.14. Remission, defined as a period of at least 12 months without any actively inflamed joints, was documented in 17.6% of patients in one study. Patients who achieved remission tended to have a lower number of actively inflamed joints at presentation [68]. Patients who sustained remission tended to be male, with a lower number of actively inflamed joints at presentation. However, after a period of remission of 2.6 years, 52% of the patients went on to flare. Only six patients sustained a complete remission, having no evidence of actively inflamed joints or damaged joints, and on no medications. ACR, American College of Rheumatology; FCI, Functional Class Index; IA, intra-articular; PASI, Psoriasis Activity and Severity Index. Adapted from [68].

HLA gene complex - chromosome 6

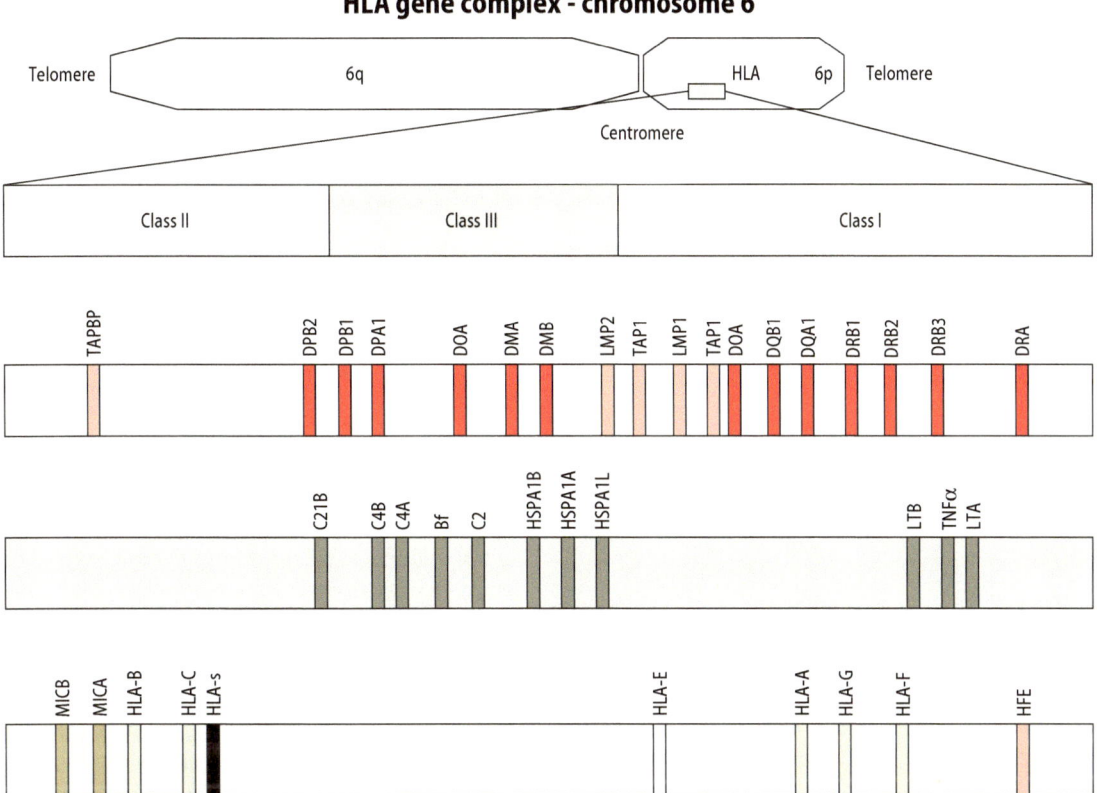

FIGURE 1.15. Human leukocyte antigen (HLA) studies support the genetic susceptibility to PsA. Class I antigens HLA-B13, HLA-B17 and its split HLA-B57, HLA-B39, HLA-Cw6, and HLA-Cw7 have consistently shown a positive association with psoriasis in population studies [69,70]. The largest and most consistently reported relative risk (RR) has been with HLA-Cw6 (RR = 22). The presence of HLA-Cw*0602 is associated with more severe psoriasis [71]. Whether the HLA-Cw*0602 allele or a neighboring gene is the susceptibility gene has yet to be determined [72]. With respect to class II antigens, HLA-DR4 and HLA-DR7 have been shown to be associated with psoriasis [73,74]. Antigens HLA-B13, HLA-B16 and its splits HLA-B38 and HLA-B39, as well as HLA-B17 and HLA-Cw6 are associated with psoriasis, with or without arthritis, while HLA-B27 and HLA-B7 are associated with PsA [69]. HLA-B27 was associated with back involvement, while HLA-B38 and HLA-B39 occurred more frequently among patients with peripheral polyarthritis [69,70,74,76]. Patients with PsA with the RA-like symmetric poly-arthritis were noted to have a higher frequency of HLA-DR4 [69]. Molecular techniques using restriction fragment length polymorphism (RFLP) analysis of class II as well as T-cell receptor genes in PsA and psoriasis demonstrated an association with the HLA-DRB1*0701 (DR7a) gene but not with T-cell receptor genes [77]. HLA-DRB1*0401 was significantly lower among patients with PsA compared with those with RA, whereas HLA-DRB1*0402 is higher among patients with PsA ($p < 0.01$) [78]. HLA-DRB1 'shared epitope' alleles were associated with radiographic changes in patients with PsA in one study [79]. MICA (MHC class I chain related), which resides centromeric to the HLA-B locus, has been found to be associated with PsA [80]. There is also evidence that other genes in the HLA region on chromosome 6 may be important, including tumor necrosis factor (TNF)-α and its promoter [81,82]. HLA has been identified as a candidate gene for PsA using sibpair analysis [83].

HLA antigens and disease progression in PsA

	Relative risk			p value
Damage state	1–2	2–3	3–4	
HLA antigen				
B22	0.19	0.19	0.19	0.002
B27	1.24	1.24	1.24	0.250
B27 x DR7	2.41	2.41	2.41	0.006
B39	6.49	2.05	1.31	<0.0001*
DR7	0.85	0.85	0.85	0.45
DQw3	1.60	1.60	1.60	0.008
DQw3 x DR7	0.51	0.51	0.51	0.032

Damage states are based on clinical features including
deformities, ankylosis, subluxation, flail joints.
1, no damage; 2, 1–4 damaged joints; 3, 5–9 damaged joints;
4, >10 damaged joints. *Applies to the 1 to 2 transition only.

FIGURE 1.16. In addition to being associated with the disease, HLAs have been identified as prognostic markers for the progression of clinical damage in PsA. In a study that included only the HLA antigens previously associated with either psoriasis or PsA, HLA antigens served as prognostic factors in patients with PsA [84]. HLA-B39 alone, HLA-B27 in the presence of HLA-DR7, and HLA-DQw3 in the absence of HLA-DR7, conferred an increased risk for disease progression measured by the extent of clinical damage. The interaction between HLA-B27 and HLA-DQw3 with HLA-DR7 suggests a role for more than one gene in disease progression. The addition of all HLA antigens detected in the patient population studied to the above model identified HLA-B22 as 'protective' for disease progression [84]. These studies used the progression of clinical damage as an outcome. The role of HLA markers in predicting progression of radiographic damage requires further study. HLA-Cw*0602 was associated with an earlier age of onset of psoriasis in patients with PsA [86]. Adapted from [84].

Genetic basis of psoriasis: genome scans

17q	Tomfohrdre J et al. Science 1994; **264**:1141–1145 [87]
	Nair RP et al. Hum Mol Genet 1997; **6**:1349–1356 [88]
4q	Matthews D et al. Nat Genet 1996; **13**:231–233 [89]
6p	Burden AD et al. Br J Dermatol 1996; **135**:815–851 [90]
	Trembath RC et al. Hum Mol Genet 1997; **6**:813–820 [91]
	Samuelsson L et al.Hum Genet 1999; **105**:523–529 [92]
	Leder RO et al. Hum Heredity 1998; **48**:198–211 [93]
	Veal CD et al. J Med Genet 2001; **38**:7–13 [94]
1p	Veal CD et al. J Med Genet 2001; **38**:7–13 [94]

FIGURE 1.17. Several genome scans performed in psoriasis have demonstrated linkage with genes on chromosome 1p, 4q, 6p, 16q, and 17q [87–94]. By far the strongest association is with a locus on chromosome 6p. Indeed, a gene for psoriasis has been proposed for that, telomeric to the HLA-B locus. A recent analysis of all families for whom complete data were available in the literature suggests that the HLA-B locus is in linkage disequilibrium with the *PSORS1* gene [93]. This gene may be the corneodesmosin gene or may be a gene close to it [95–97]. Most recently, the International Psoriasis Genetics Consortium assessed linkage to 14 candidate genes previously reported in psoriasis [98]. They confirmed the strong linkage with the MHC, and evidence for allele sharing on chromosomes 16q and 10q. The studies in this figure included primarily patients with psoriasis, with minimal analysis of patients with PsA. A recent study documented a locus for PsA on 16q [99]. The peak of the LOD score is within 20 Mb of the *CARD15* gene (MIM 605956), similar to the area implicated from a genome-wide scan in psoriasis [88]. *CARD15* has been shown to confer susceptibility to Crohn's disease [100], where there is an increased incidence of psoriasis. Although no association between CARD15 polymorphisms and psoriasis was detected in two studies [101,102], *CARD15* was recently found to be an independent non-HLA gene associated with PsA [103]. This latter study was performed in a founder population in Newfoundland, Canada, and may reflect linkage disequilibrium with another gene that has yet to be identified. Thus, while there are some genetic factors that predispose to both psoriasis and PsA, others are identified for specific manifestations of the disease.

References

1. Wright V, Moll JMH. **Psoriatic arthritis.** *Bull Rheum Dis* 1971; 21:627–632.
2. Wright V. **Rheumatism and psoriasis: a re-evaluation.** *Am J Med* 1959; 27:454–462.
3. Gladman DD. **Classification criteria for psoriatic arthritis.** *Baillieres Clin Rheumatol* 1995; 9:319–329.
4. Taylor WJ, Gladman DD, Helliwell PS *et al.* **Classification criteria for psoriatic arthritis.** *Arthritis Rheum* 2006; 54:2665–2673.
5. Schentag CT, Cichon J, MacKinnon A *et al.* **Validation and normative data for the 0–10 point scale version of the fatigue severity scale (FSS).** *Arthritis Rheum* 2000; 43(Suppl 9):S177.
6. Schentag CT, Beaton M, Rahman P *et al.* **Prevalence and correlates of fatigue in psoriatic arthritis (PsA).** *Arthritis Rheum* 2000; 43(Suppl 9):S105.
7. Schentag C, Gladman DD. **Changes in fatigue in psoriatic arthritis: Disease activity or fibromyalgia.** *Arthritis Rheum* 2002; 46(Suppl 9):S424.
8. Chandran V, Bhella S, Schentag C *et al.* **Functional assessment of chronic illness therapy fatigues scale in psoriatic arthritis: a validation study.** *Ann Rheum Dis* 2006; 65(Suppl II):210.
9. Mease PJ, Gladman DD, Ritchlin CT *et al.* Adalimumab Effectiveness in Psoriatic Arthritis Trial Study Group. **Adalimumab for the treatment of patients with moderately to severely active psoriatic arthritis: results of a double-blind, randomized, placebo-controlled trial.** *Arthritis Rheum* 2005; 52:3279–3289.
10. Brockbank JE, Schentag CT, Gladman DD. **Musculo-skeletal and cutaneous disease in the parents of patients with psoriatic arthritis (PsA).** *Arthritis Rheum* 2003; 48(Suppl 9):S603.
11. Brandrup F, Holm N, Grunnet N *et al.* **Psoriasis in monozygotic twins: variations in expression in individuals with identical genetic constitution.** *Acta Dermato-Venereol* 1982; 62:229–236.
12. Farber EM, Nall L, Watson W. **Natural history of psoriasis in 61 twin pairs.** *Arch Dermatol* 1974; 109:207–211.
13. Watson W, Cann HM. **The genetics of psoriasis.** *Arch Dermatol* 1972; 105:197–207.
14. Pedersen OB, Svendsen AJ, Ejstrup L *et al.* **Two Danish twin studies in psoriatic arthritis.** *Arthritis Rheum* 2004; 50(Suppl 9):S215.
15. Bhalerao J, Bowcock AM. **The genetics of psoriasis: a complex disorder of the skin and immune system.** *Hum Mol Genet* 1998; 7:1537–1545.
16. Moll JM, Wright V. **Familial occurrence of PsA.** *Ann Rheum Dis* 1973; 32:181–201.
17. Risch N. **Linkage strategies for genetically complex traits. 1. Multilocus model.** *Am J Hum Genet* 1990; 46:222–228.
18. O'Neill T, Silman AJ. **Psoriatic arthritis. Historical background and epidemiology.** *Baillieres Clin Rheumatol* 1994; 8:245–261.
19. Kaipiainen-Seppanen O. **Incidence of psoriatic arthritis in Finland.** *Br J Rheumatol* 1996; 35:1289–1291.
20. Shbeeb M, Uramoto KM, Gibson LE *et al.* **The epidemiology of psoriatic arthritis in Olmsted County, Minnesota, USA, 1982–1991.** *J Rheumatol* 2000; 27:1247–1250.
21. Hukuda S, Minami M, Saito T *et al.* **Spondyloarthropathies in Japan: nationwide questionnaire survey performed by the Japan Ankylosing Spondylitis Society.** *J Rheumatol* 2001; 28:554–559.
22. Soderlin MK, Borjesson O, Kautiainen H *et al.* **Annual incidence of inflammatory joint diseases in a population based study in southern Sweden.** *Ann Rheum Dis* 2002; 61:911–915.
23. Savolainen E, Kaipiainen-Seppanen O, Kroger L *et al.* **Total incidence and distribution of inflammatory joint diseases in a defined population: results from the Kuopio 2000 arthritis survey.** *J Rheumatol* 2003; 30:2460–2468.
24. Alamanos Y, Papadopoulos NG, Voulgari PV *et al.* **Epidemiology of psoriatic arthritis in northwest Greece, 1982–2001.** *J Rheumatol* 2003; 30:2641–2644.
25. Minaur N, Sawyers S, Parker J *et al.* **Rheumatic disease in an Australian Aboriginal community in North Queensland, Australia. A WHO-ILAR COPCORD survey.** *J Rheumatol* 2004; 31:965–972.
26. Gorter S, van der Heijde DM, van der Linden S *et al.* **Psoriatic arthritis: performance of rheumatologists in daily practice.** *Ann Rheum Dis* 2002; 61:219–224.
27. Leczinsky CG. **The incidence of arthropathy in a ten-year series of psoriasis cases.** *Acta Derm Venereol* 1948; 28:483–487.
28. Vilanova X, Pinol J. **Psoriasis arthropathica.** *Rheumatism* 1951; 7:197–208.
29. Little H, Harvie JN, Lester RS. **Psoriatic arthritis in severe psoriasis.** *Can Med Assoc J* 1975;112:317–319.
30. Scarpa R, Oriente P, Pucino A *et al.* **Psoriatic arthritis in psoriatic patients.** *Br J Rheumatol* 1984; 23:246–250.
31. Stern RS. **The epidemiology of joint complaints in patients with psoriasis.** *J Rheumatol* 1985; 12:315–320.
32. Zanelli MD, Wilde JS. **Joint complaints in psoriasis patients.** *Int J Dermatol* 1992; 31:488–491.

33. Barišic-Druško V, Dobric I, Paic A *et al.* **Frequency of psoriatic arthritis in general population and among psoriatics in department of dermatology.** *Acta Derm Venerol (Stockh)* 1994; **74**(Suppl 186): 107–108.

34. Salvarani C, Lo Scocco G, Macchioni P *et al.* **Prevalence of psoriatic arthritis in Italian patients with psoriasis.** *J Rheumatol* 1995; **22**:1499–1503.

35. Shbeeb M, Uramoto KM, Gibson LE *et al.* **The epidemiology of psoriatic arthritis in Olmsted County, Minnesota, USA, 1982–1991.** *J Rheumatol* 2000; **27**:1247–1250.

36. Brockbank JE, Schentag C, Rosen C *et al.* **Psoriatic arthritis (PsA) is common among patients with psoriasis and family medical clinic attendees.** *Arthritis Rheum* 2001; **44**(Suppl 9):S94.

37. Alenius GM, Stenberg B, Stenlund H *et al.* **Inflammatory joint manifestations are prevalent in psoriasis: prevalence study of joint and axial involvement in psoriatic patients, and evaluation of a psoriatic and arthritic questionnaire.** *J Rheumatol* 2002; **29**:2577–2582.

38. Zachariae H. **Prevalence of joint disease in patients with psoriasis: implications for therapy.** *Am J Clin Dermatol* 2003; **4**:441–447.

39. Trabace S, Cappellacci S, Ciccarone P *et al.* **Psoriatic arthritis: a clinical, radiological and genetic study of 58 Italian patients.** *Acta Derm Venereol* 1994; **186**:69–70.

40. Marsal S, Armadans-Gil L, Martinez M *et al.* **Clinical, radiographic and HLA associations as markers for different patterns of psoriatic arthritis.** *Rheumatology* 1999; **38**:332–337.

41. Torre Alonso JC, Rodriguez Perez A, Arribas Castrillo JM *et al.* **Psoriatic arthritis (PA): a clinical, immunological and radiological study of 180 patients.** *Br J Rheumatol* 1991; **30**:245–250.

42. Gladman DD, Shuckett R, Russell ML *et al.* **Psoriatic arthritis (PSA) – an analysis of 220 patients.** *Q J Med* 1987; **62**:127–141.

43. Jones SM, Armas JB, Cohen MG *et al.* **Psoriatic arthritis: outcome of disease subsets and relationship of joint disease to nail and skin disease.** *Br J Rheumatol* 1984; **33**:834–839.

44. Helliwell P, Marchesoni A, Peters M *et al.* **A re-evaluation of the osteoarticular manifestations of psoriasis.** *Br J Rheumatol* 1991; **30**:339–345.

45. Veale D, Rogers S, Fitzgerald O. **Classification of clinical subsets in psoriatic arthritis.** *Br J Rheumatol* 1994; **33**:133–138.

46. Jones SM, Armas JB, Cohen MG *et al.* **Psoriatic arthritis: outcome of disease subsets and relationship of joint disease to nail and skin disease.** *Br J Rheumatol* 1994; **33**:834–839.

47. Kane D, Stafford L, Bresnihan B *et al.* **A classification study of clinical subsets in an inception cohort of early psoriatic peripheral arthritis – 'DIP or not DIP revisited'.** *Rheumatology* 2003; **42**:1469–1476.

48. Khan M, Schentag C, Gladman D. **Clinical and radiological changes during psoriatic arthritis disease progression: Working toward classification criteria.** *J Rheumatol* 2003; **30**:1022–1026.

49. Gladman DD, Brubacher B, Buskila D *et al.* **Psoriatic spondyloarthropathy in men and women: A clinical, radiographic and HLA study.** *Clin Invest Med* 1992; **15**:371–375.

50. McHorney CA, Ware JE Jr, Lu JF *et al.* **The MOS 36-item Short-Form Health Survey (SF-36): III. Tests of data quality, scaling assumptions, and reliability across diverse patient groups.** *Med Care* 1994; **32**:40–66.

51. Husted JA, Gladman DD, Farewell VT *et al.* **Validating the SF-36 health survey questionnaire in patients with psoriatic arthritis.** *J Rheumatol* 1997; **24**:511–517.

52. Husted JA, Gladman DD, Cook RJ *et al.* **Responsiveness of health status instruments to changes in articular status and perceived health in patients with psoriatic arthritis (PsA).** *J Rheumatol* 1998; **25**:2146–2155.

53. McKenna SP, Doward LC, Whalley D *et al.* **Development of the PsAQoL: a quality of life instrument specific to psoriatic arthritis.** *Ann Rheum* 2004; **63**:162–169.

54. Husted JA, Gladman DD, Farewell VT *et al.* **Health-related quality of life of patients with psoriatic arthritis: a comparison with patients with rheumatoid arthritis.** *Arthritis Rheum* 2001; **45**:151–158.

55. Sokoll KB, Helliwell PS. **Comparison of disability and quality of life in rheumatoid and psoriatic arthritis.** *J Rheumatol* 2001; **28**:1842–1846.

56. Mease PJ, Kivitz AJ, Burch FX *et al.* **Etanercept treatment of psoriatic arthritis: safety, efficacy, and effect on disease progression.** *Arthritis Rheum* 2004; **50**:2264–2272.

57. Antoni C, Krueger GG, de Vlam K *et al.* **Infliximab improves signs and symptoms of psoriatic arthritis: results of the IMPACT 2 trial.** *Ann Rheum Dis* 2005; **64**:1150–1157.

58. Mease PJ, Ganguly R, Wanke L *et al.* **How much improvement in functional status is considered important by patients with active psoriatic arthritis: applying the outcome measures in rheumatoid arthritis clinical trials (OMERACT) group guidelines.** *Ann Rheum Dis* 2004; **63**(Suppl 1):391.

59. Coulton BL, Thomson K, Symmons DPM *et al*. **Outcome in patients hospitalised for psoriatic arthritis**. *Clin Rheumatol* 1989; 2:261–265.

60. Gladman DD. **The natural history of psoriatic arthritis**. In: *Baillière's Clinical Rheumatology. International Practice and Research*. Edited by V Wright, P Helliwell. London: Baillière Tindall; 1994; 379–394.

61. McHugh NJ, Balachrishnan C, Jones SM. **Progression of peripheral joint disease in psoriatic arthritis: a 5-yr prospective study**. *Rheumatology* 2003; 42:778–783.

62. Gladman DD, Farewell VT, Nadeau C. **Clinical indicators of progression in psoriatic arthritis (PSA): multivariate relative risk model**. *J Rheumatol* 1995; 22:675–679.

63. Gladman DD, Farewell VT, Kopciuk K *et al*. **HLA antigens and progression in psoriatic arthritis**. *J Rheumatol* 1998; 25:730–733.

64. Queiro-Silva R, Torre-Alonso JC, Tinture-Eguren T *et al*. **A polyarticular onset predicts erosive and deforming disease in psoriatic arthritis**. *Ann Rheum Dis* 2003; 62:68–70.

65. Kane D, Stafford L, Bresniham B *et al*. **A prospective, clinical and radiological study of early psoriatic arthritis: an early synovitis clinic experience**. *Rheumatology* 2003; 42:1460–1468.

66. Wong K, Gladman DD, Husted J *et al*. **Mortality studies in psoriatic arthritis: results from a single centre. I. Risk and causes of death**. *Arthritis Rheum* 1997; 40:1868–1872.

67. Gladman DD, Farewell VT, Wong K *et al*. **Mortality studies in psoriatic arthritis: results from a single centre. II. Prognostic indicators for death**. *Arthritis Rheum* 1998; 41:1103–1110.

68. Gladman DD, Hing EN, Schentag CT *et al*. **Remission in psoriatic arthritis**. *J Rheumatol* 2001; 28:1045–1048.

69. Gladman DD, Anhorn KAB, Schachter RK *et al*. **HLA antigens in PsA**. *J Rheumatol* 1986; 13:586–592.

70. Eastmond CJ. **Genetics and HLA antigens**. In: *Ballière's Clinical Rheumatology. Psoriatic Arthritis*. Edited by V Wright, P Helliwell. London: Ballière Tindall, 1994; 263–276.

71. Guojonsson JE, Karason A, Antonsdottir AA *et al*. **HLA-Cw6-positive and HLA-Cw6-negative patients with psoriasis vulgaris have distinct clinical features**. *J Invest Dermatol* 2002; 118:362–365.

72. Oka A, Tamiya G, Tmozawa M *et al*. **Association analysis using refined microsatellite markers localizes a susceptibility locus for psoriasis vulgaris within a 111 kb segment telomeric of the HLA-C gene**. Hum Mol Genet 1999; 8:2165–2170.

73. Russell TJ, Schultes LM, Kuban DJ. **Histocompatibility (HL-A) antigens associated with psoriasis**. *N Engl J Med* 1972; 287:738–743.

74. Tiwari JL, Lowe NJ, Abramovits W *et al*. **Association of psoriasis with HLA-DR7**. *Br J Dermatol* 1982; 106:227–230.

75. Espinoza LR, Vasey FB, Gaylord SW *et al*. **Histocompatibility typing in the seronegative spondyloarthropathies: a survey**. *Semin Arthritis Rheum* 1982; 11:375–381.

76. Salvarani C, Macchioni PL, Zizzi F *et al*. **Clinical subgroups in Italian patients with psoriatic arthritis**. *Clin Exp Rheumatol* 1989; 7:391–396.

77. Sakkas LI, Loqueman N, Bird H *et al*. **HLA class II and T cell receptor gene polymorphism in psoriatic arthritis and psoriasis**. *J Rheumatol* 1990; 17:1487–1490.

78. Gladman DD, Farewell VT, Rahman P *et al*. **HLA-DRB1*04 alleles in psoriatic arthritis (PsA): comparison with rheumatoid arthritis and healthy controls**. *Hum Immunol* 2001; 62:1239–1244.

79. Korendowych E, Dixey J, Cox B *et al*. **The Influence of the HLA-DRB1 rheumatoid arthritis shared epitope on the clinical characteristics and radiological outcome of psoriatic arthritis**. *J Rheumatol* 2003; 30:96–101.

80. Gonzalez S, Martinez-Borra J, Torre-Alonso JC *et al*. **The MIC-A9 triplet repeat polymorphism in the transmembrane region confers additional susceptibility to develop psoriatic arthritis, and is independent of the association of Cw*602 in psoriasis**. *Arthritis Rheum* 1999; 42:1010–1016.

81. Al-Heresh AM, Proctor J, Jones SM *et al*. **Tumour necrosis factor-α polymorphisms and the HLA-Cw*602 allele in psoriatic arthritis**. *Rheumatology* 2002; 41:525–530.

82. Hohler T, Grossmann S, Stradmann-Bellinghausen B *et al*. **Differential association of polymorphisms in the TNFα region with psoriatic arthritis but not psoriasis**. *Ann Rheum Dis* 2002; 61:213–218.

83. Gladman DD, Farewell VT, Pellett F *et al*. **HLA is a candidate region for psoriatic arthritis: Evidence for excessive HLA sharing in sibling pairs**. *Hum Immunol* 2003; 64:887–889.

84. Gladman DD, Farewell VT. **The role of HLA antigens as indicators of progression in psoriatic arthritis (PsA): multivariate relative risk model**. *Arthritis Rheum* 1995; 38:845–850.

85. Gladman DD, Farewell VT, Kopciuk K *et al*. **HLA antigens and progression in psoriatic arthritis**. *J Rheumatol* 1998; 25:730–733.

86. Gladman DD, Cheung C, Ng CM et al. HLA C-locus alleles in psoriatic arthritis (PsA). Hum Immunol 1999; 60:259–261.

87. Tomfohrdre J, Silverman A, Barnes R et al. Gene for familial psoriasis susceptibility mapped to the distal end of human chromosome 17q. Science 1994; 264:1141–1145.

88. Nair RP, Henseler T, Jenisch S et al. Evidence for two psoriasis susceptibility loci (HLA and 17q) and two novel candidate regions (16q and 20p) by genome-wide scan. Hum Mol Genet 1997; 6:1349–1356.

89. Matthews D, Fry L, Powles A et al. Evidence that a locus for familial psoriasis maps to chromosome 4q. Nat Genet 1996; 13:231–233.

90. Burden AD, Javed S, Hodgins M et al. Linkage to chromosome 6p and exclusion of chromosome 17q in familial psoriasis in Scotland. Br J Dermatol 1996; 135:815–851.

91. Trembath RC, Clough RL, Rosbotham JL et al. Identification of a major susceptibility locus on chromosome 6p an evidence for further disease loci revealed by two stage genome-wide search in psoriasis. Hum Mol Genet 1997; 6:813–820.

92. Samuelsson L, Enlund F, Torinsson A et al. A genome-wide search for genes predisposing to familial psoriasis by using a stratification approach. Hum Genet 1999; 105:523–529.

93. Leder RO, Mansbridge JN, Hallmayer J et al. Familial psoriasis and HLA-B: Unambiguous support for linkage in 97 published families. Hum Heredity 1998; 48:198–211.

94. Veal CD, Clough RL, Barber RC et al. Identification of a novel psoriasis susceptibility locus at 1p and evidence of epistasis between PSORSI and candidate loci. J Med Genet 2001; 38:7–13.

95. Schmitt-Egenolf M, Windemuth C, Hennies HC et al. Comparative association analysis reveals that corneodesmosin is more closely associated with psoriasis than HLA-Cw*0602B*5701 in German families. Tissue Antigens 2001; 57:440–446.

96. Elder JT, Nair RP, Henseler T et al. The genetics of psoriasis 2001. The odyssey continues. Arch Dermatol 2001; 137:1447–1454.

97. Orrù S, Giuressi E, Casual M et al. Psoriasis is associated with a SNP haplotype of the corneodesmosin gene (CDSN). Tissue Antigens 2002; 60:292–298.

98. The international psoriasis genetics study: Assessing linkage to 14 candidate susceptibility loci in a cohort of 942 affected sib pairs. Am J Hum Genet 2003; 73:430–437.

99. Karason A, Gudjonsson JE, Upmanyu R et al. A susceptibility gene for psoriatic arthritis maps to chromosome 16q: evidence for imprinting. Am J Hum Genet 2003; 72:125–131.

100. Hugot JP, Chamaillard M, Zouali H et al. Association of NOD2 leucine-rich repeat variants with susceptibility to Crohn's disease. Nature 2001; 411:599–603.

101. Nair RP, Stuart P, Ogura Y et al. Lack of association between NOD2 3020 InsC frameshift mutation and psoriasis. J Invest Dermatol 2001; 117:1671–1672.

102. Borgiani P, Vallo L, D'Apice MR et al. Exclusion of CARD15/NOD2 as a candidate susceptibility gene to psoriasis in the Italian population. Eur J Dermatol 2002; 12:540–542.

103. Rahman P, Bartlett S, Farewell VT et al. CARD15: a pleiotropic autoimmune gene – a susceptibility gene for psoriatic arthritis. Am J Human Genet 2003; 73:677–681.

2
Etiology and Pathophysiology

Christopher Ritchlin and Jennifer Barton

Initially considered to be relatively benign and uncommon, one-third of patients with psoriasis have arthritis, and a majority of those affected experience a chronic, progressive course [1,2]. Psoriatic arthritis (PsA) is distinguished from rheumatoid arthritis (RA) by its unique clinical manifestations, characteristic radiographic findings, and the absence of rheumatoid factor. Patients often present with focal inflammation at multiple sites that include skin, joints, and tendon insertion sites or entheses. Clues to the pathogenesis of the disease have arisen out of observations that reveal a strong family history of psoriasis in PsA patients, an association of skin and joint disease with class I major histocompatibility complex (MHC) alleles, and paternal transmission. Environmental factors such as trauma or infection have also been shown to trigger skin and joint inflammation. The uncovering of the pathogenesis of PsA has been limited by small numbers of studies, the paucity of appropriate animal models, and the confounding presence of a disease within a disease, whereby factors associated with psoriasis can obscure those related to arthritis. However, the advent of biological therapies has improved treatment responses and helped to further the understanding of the role of specific effector cell populations to ongoing inflammation and to better define the role of both pro- and anti-inflammatory cytokines *in vivo*. This chapter will review the etiology of PsA, including a discussion of genetic and environmental factors, as well as the pathophysiology of the four principle anatomic sites of involvement in the disease: psoriatic plaque, the synovial membrane, the enthesis, and bony and cartilaginous structures in the psoriatic joint.

Etiology

Genetic factors

Population and twin studies support the influence of heritable factors on phenotypic expression of psoriasis and PsA [3]. (*See* Chapter 1, *Epidemiology*, for a detailed discussion of the role of genetics in PsA.)

Environmental factors

Compelling evidence suggests that trauma and infection play a prominent role in the etiologic pathway of PsA. Koebner phenomenon (psoriatic lesions arising at sites of trauma) occurs in up to one-quarter to one-half of psoriasis patients [4]. In one study, 25% of patients reported development of PsA following trauma to a joint.

Infection has been linked to PsA. In children, a strikingly high association between guttate psoriasis and preceding streptococcal pharyngitis and tonsillitis exists [5]. In adults, circulating antibodies to microbial peptidoglycans and elevated levels of group A streptococcal 16S RNA have been identified in the blood of PsA patients, but not in controls [6]. The striking inflammatory response to streptococcal and staphylococcal superantigens in non-involved psoriatic skin, but not in atopic dermatitis or lichen planus, suggests that superantigen pathways of cell activation may be important in psoriasis [7,8].

Pathogenesis

Traditionally, psoriasis has been viewed as a hyper-proliferative disorder [9]. Initial research efforts focused on abnormal keratinocyte proliferation. More recently, emphasis has shifted to the role of T-lymphocytes as the critical effector cells necessary for the induction of psoriasis. Evidence from the severe combined immunodeficiency (SCID) mouse:human skin chimera model and from reports showing the effect of specific anti-T-cell therapies (cyclosporine, 6-thioguanine, and diphtheria IL-2 fusion toxin) in psoriasis have underscored the importance of these cells in the disease [10].

Synovial membrane characteristics

Several histopathologic features appear to distinguish PsA from RA. In one study, the degree of lymphocytic infiltration was similar, but the psoriatic synovial tissues showed greater vascularity and less synovial lining hyperplasia and monocyte/macrophage infiltration than rheumatoid tissues [11]. A striking feature seen in psoriatic but not rheumatoid joints, when viewed through an arthroscope, is the marked tortuosity and dilatation of blood vessels [12]. Levels of vascular endothelial growth factor (VEGF) and angiopoietin-2 (Ang-2) were upregulated in psoriatic compared with rheumatoid synovium in early disease; methotrexate reduced tissue vascularity and VEGF levels [13]. Higher levels of helper T-lymphocyte cytokines IL-2 and interferon-gamma were produced in tissue explants from psoriatic when compared with rheumatoid patients [14].

Enthesis

Unusual in RA, enthesopathy or inflammation at tendon or ligamentous insertion sites is a hallmark feature of PsA [15]. Most common clinical syndromes include plantar fasciitis, epicondylitis, and Achilles tendonitis. Pathogenesis of enthesopathy is not well understood but fat-suppressed magnetic resonance imaging (MRI) studies reveal bone marrow edema adjacent to entheseal insertion sites [16] and, on biopsy, infiltration of CD8 cells and macrophages in underlying subchondral bone [17]. Treatment with an anti-tumor necrosis factor (TNF) agent, etanercept, reversed abnormal MRI signals [18].

Mechanisms of joint destruction

Radiographs of psoriatic joints often manifest cartilage loss through joint space narrowing as well as altered bone remodeling as seen in the form of tuft resorption, large eccentric erosions, and pencil-in-cup deformities. Cartilage destruction is mediated by matrix metalloproteinases (MMPs), enzymes that degrade collagens and other matrix molecules (proteoglycans, fibronectin, gelatins, laminin). MMP-1 to MMP-3 and MMP-9 have been detected in PsA synovium. In addition, tissue inhibitors of metalloproteinases (TIMP-1, TIMP-2) have been identified in cells infiltrating the psoriatic synovial lining.

Psoriatic joint biopsies demonstrate large multinucleated osteoclasts in deep resorption pits at the bone-pannus junction [19]. Osteoclastogenesis (differentiation of osteoclasts) is a contact-dependent process [20]. Osteoblasts and stromal cells in the bone marrow direct this process by release of two different signals (macrophage-colony-stimulating factor [M-CSF] and receptor activator of NF-κ B ligand [RANKL]) that stimulate proliferation and differentiation of an osteoclast precursor (OCP) [21]. Osteoprotegerin (OPG) is the natural antagonist of RANKL [22].

In psoriatic synovial tissues, marked upregulation of RANKL protein and low expression of OPG was detected in the adjacent synovial lining. OCPs were also noted to be markedly elevated in the peripheral blood of PsA patients compared with healthy controls [19]. Treatment of PsA patients with anti-TNF agents significantly decreased levels of OCPs. New bone formation manifests radiographically as periostitis and bony ankylosis [23]. The cellular and molecular mechanisms that are responsible for new bone formation are unknown, although a role for VEGF and bone morphogenic protein (BMP)-4 has been proposed [24].

Environmental factors in the pathogenesis of RA

Trauma	Koebner phenomenon (psoriatic lesions arising at sites of trauma) occurs in up to a quarter to one-half of PsA patients. PsA has also been reported to arise in joints subjected to trauma (deep Koebner phenomenon)
Infection	In children, a strikingly high association between guttate psoriasis and preceding streptococcal pharyngitis and tonsillitis exists. High levels of circulating antibodies to microbial peptidoglycans and elevated levels of group A streptococcus 16S RNA identified in peripheral blood of PsA patients [6]
	Streptococcal and staphylococcal superantigens promote inflammation and upregulate keratinocyte TNF mRNA expression when applied to non-involved psoriatic skin

FIGURE 2.1. mRNA, messenger RNA; PsA, psoriatic arthritis; RA, rheumatoid arthritis; RNA, ribonucleic acid; TNF, tumor necrosis factor.

Histology of psoriatic plaque

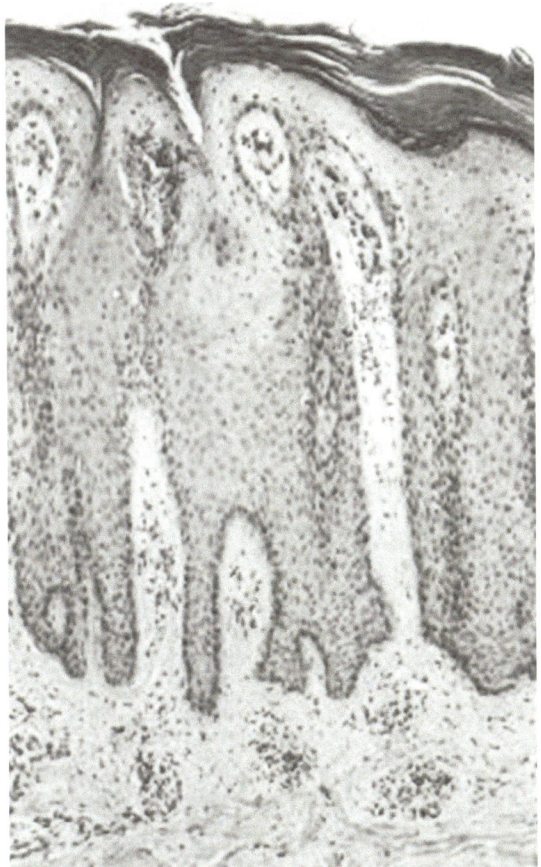

FIGURE 2.2. Note striking acanthosis (excessive thickening of the intermediate cell layer), elongation of rete-ridges, and intense subdermal perivascular lymphocytic infiltrate.

Vascular morphology in psoriatic and rheumatoid synovium

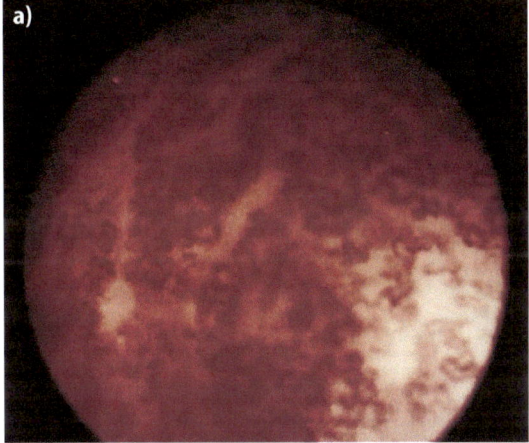

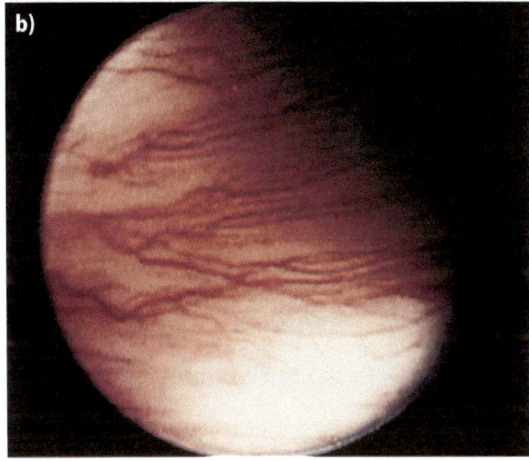

FIGURE 2.3. Vascular morphology in **(a)** psoriatic and **(b)** rheumatoid synovium as viewed through an arthroscope. Note the tortuous bushy vessels in the psoriatic membranes compared with the straight, branching pattern characteristic of rheumatoid synovium. Reproduced with permission from [12].

In situ hybridization for VEGF and Ang-2 mRNA in patients with early PsA and RA

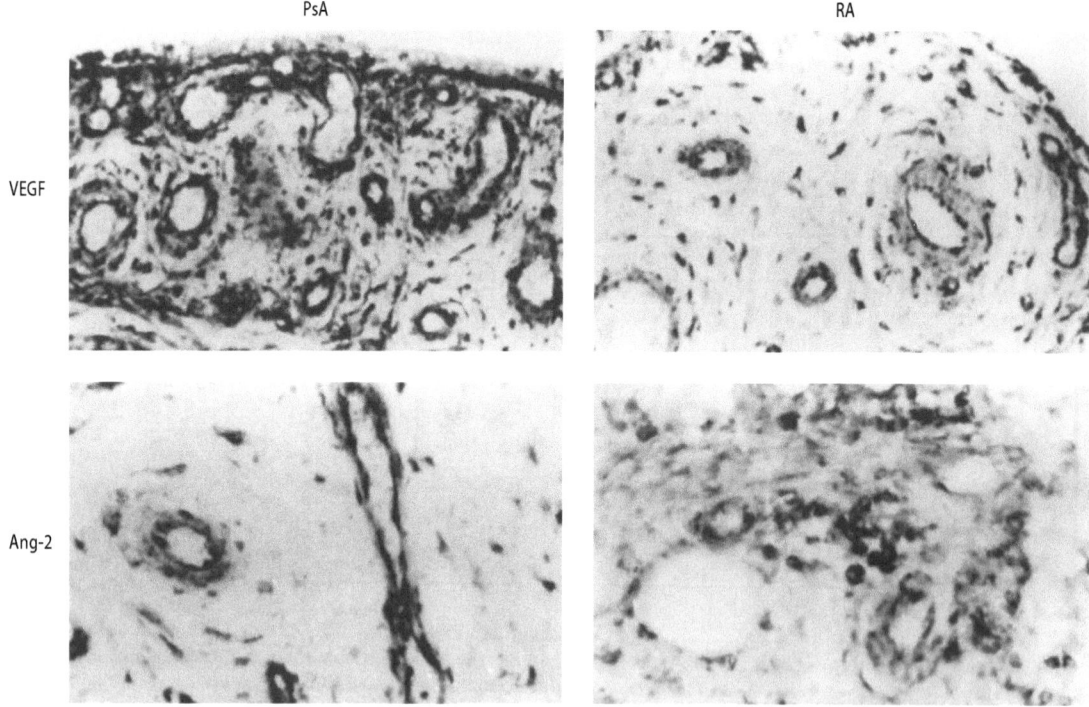

FIGURE 2.4. Synovial specimens from patients with PsA and RA were hybridized with vascular endothelial growth factor (VEGF) and angiopoietin-2 (Ang-2) mRNA probes. VEGF and Ang-2 mRNA expression were significantly higher in PsA synovial specimens. Representative synovial tissues from a PsA and RA joint are shown. Reproduced with permission from [13].

Synovial membrane characteristics – features of psoriatic synovium

Synovial lining thickness	Less synovial lining layer hyperplasia and monocyte/macrophage infiltration than rheumatoid specimens [11]
Vascularity	Marked tortuosity and dilation of blood vessels in a psoriatic joint viewed through an arthroscope [12]
	Upregulated levels of VEGF and Ang-2 compared to rheumatoid synovium in early disease [13]
Cytokines	Th1 pattern of cytokine production (IL-2 and IFN-γ but not IL-4 and IL-5) [14,25]. High concentrations of IL-10, IL-1β, and TNF-α [26,27]
T-lymphocytes	Infiltrating T-lymphocytes enter deeper layers in both psoriatic skin and joints and promote hyperproliferation of more superficial cells (keratinocytes in skin and synovial lining cells in the joint)

FIGURE 2.5. IFN, interferon; IL, interleukin; Th1, T helper 1 cell; TNF-α, tumor necrosis factor-alpha.

MRI showing acute enthesitis

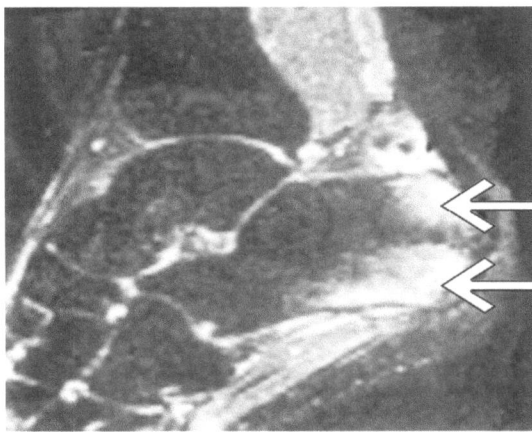

FIGURE 2.6. Magnetic resonance imaging (MRI) showing acute enthesitis in the plantar fascia and the Achilles tendon. Diffuse osteitis is seen adjacent to insertions (arrows).

Undifferentiated SpA at baseline and 6 months after treatment

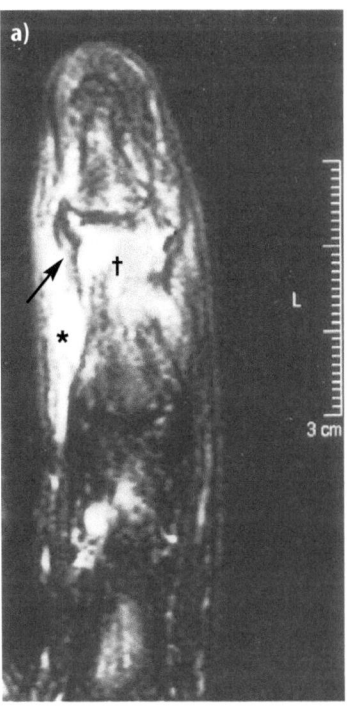 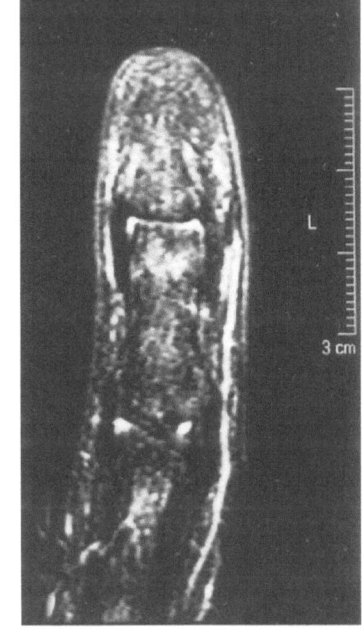

FIGURE 2.7. T1-weighted, fat-suppressed, post-gadolinium coronal sequence of the left second distal interphalangeal (DIP) joint of a patient with undifferentiated spondyloarthropathy (SpA). **(a)** Baseline study showing subcutaneous edema (asterisk) and bone marrow edema (dagger). Note inflammatory changes in the collateral ligament (black arrow). **(b)** The same joint after 6 months treatment with the anti-TNF agent etanercept. Reproduced with permission from [18].

Distal digit osteolysis in PsA

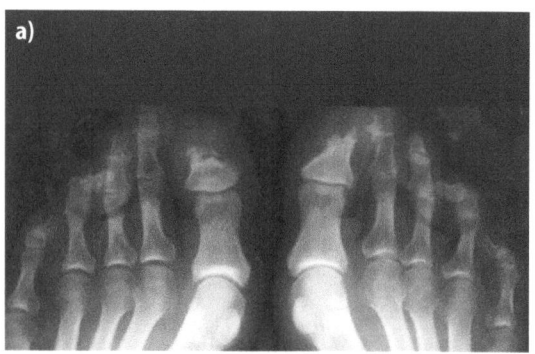
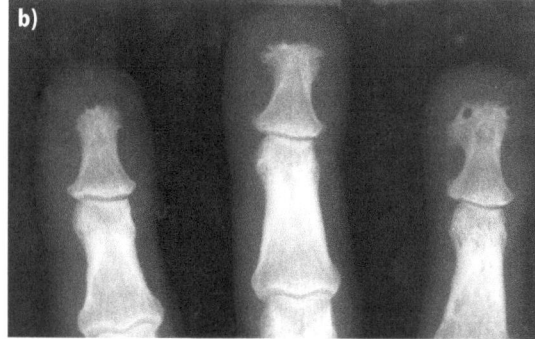

FIGURE 2.8. Osteolysis of the distal digits of **(a)** the feet and **(b)** hands of a patient with PsA. Reproduced with permission from [28].

Osteoclasts are prominent in the psoriatic joint

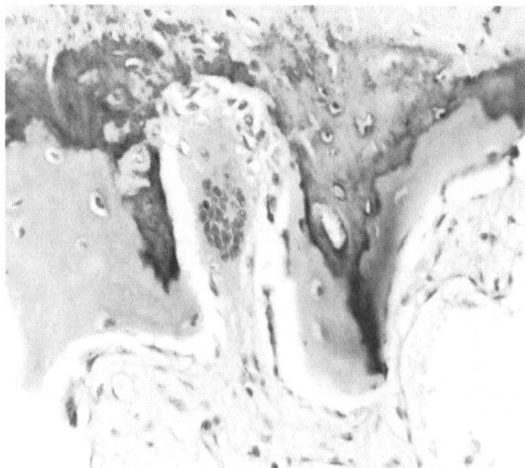

FIGURE 2.9. A representative example of a large multinucleated osteoclast at the advancing edge of the pannus in a psoriatic joint. Reproduced with permission from [19].

Bone and cartilage destruction in PsA

Radiographs	Joint space narrowing
	Altered bone remodeling • tuft resorption • large eccentric erosions • pencil-in-cup deformities
	New bone formation • periostitis • bony ankylosis [23]
Cartilage	
Matrix metalloproteinases (MMPs) and tissue inhibitors of MMPs (TIMPs)	MMP-9 localizes to blood vessel walls
	MMP-1 to MMP-3 and TIMP-1 and TIMP-2 show cellular and interstitial staining pattern in synovial lining
	MMP-3 serum levels markedly decrease following anti-TNF therapy [29,30]

FIGURE 2.10

FIGURE 2.11. (1) Osteoblasts and stromal cells express receptor activator of NF-κ B ligand (RANKL) in response to a variety of factors, including parathyroid hormone (PTH), vitamin D (vit D), and TNF-α. **(2)** RANKL binds to the receptor RANK expressed on the surface of preosteoclasts (CD14⁺ monocytes) and osteoclasts (OCs). **(3)** In the presence of monocyte-colonystimulating factor (M-CSF) and RANKL, preosteoclasts mature into OCs capable of resorbing bone. **(4)** Osteoprotegerin (OPG), a physiologic decoy molecule, can bind to RANKL and inhibit OC differentiation and activation. In the inflamed joint, synovial lining fibroblastoid cells and infiltrating T-lymphocytes express RANKL. Reproduced with permission from [31].

Osteoclastogenesis pathway

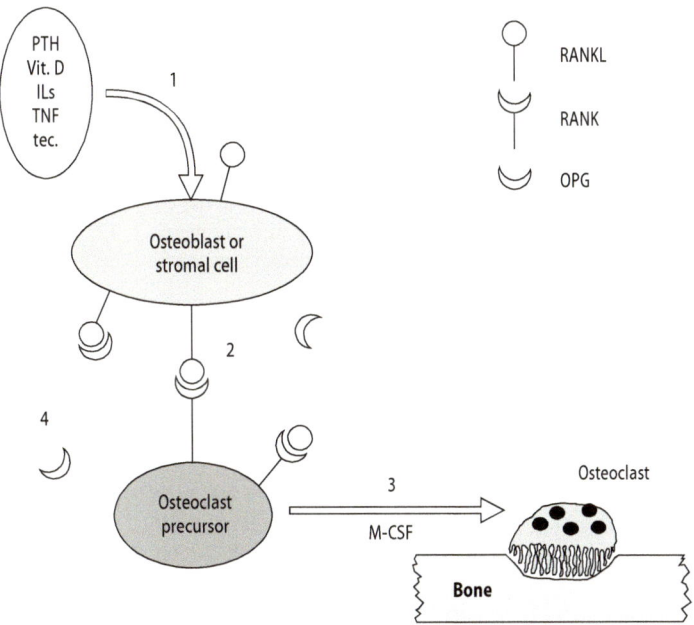

Schematic model of osteolysis in the psoriatic joint

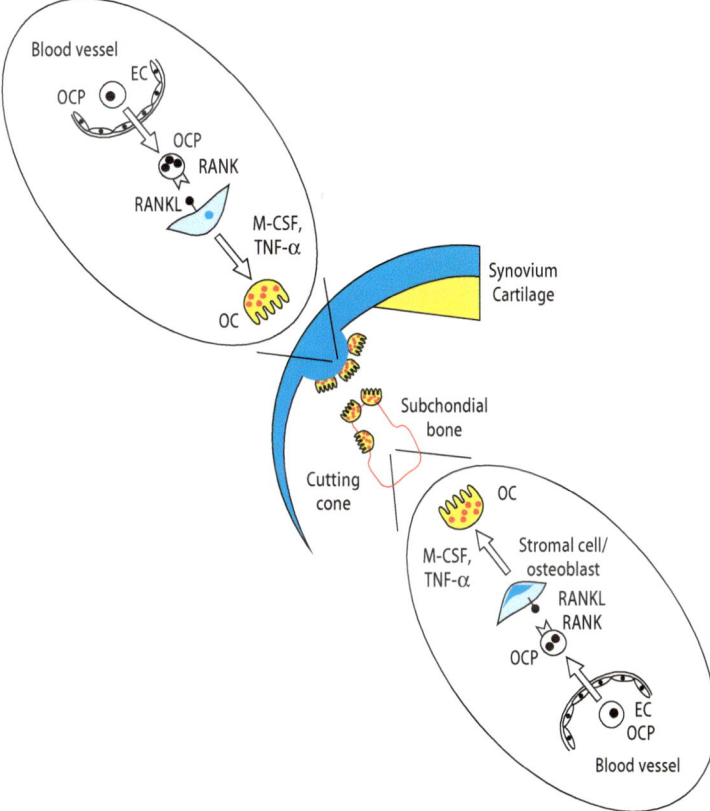

FIGURE 2.12. Extensive erosions in PsA are mediated by a bi-directional attack on bone. Circulating osteoclast precursors (OCPs) enter the synovium and are induced to become OCs by receptor activator of RANKL expressed on synoviocytes (outside–in). In parallel, OCPs traverse endothelial cells and undergo osteoclastogenesis following RANKL stimulation from osteoblasts (inside–out). EC, endothelial cell.

References

1. Alenius GM, Stenberg B, Stenlund H *et al.* **Inflammatory joint manifestations are prevalent in psoriasis: prevalence study of joint and axial involvement in psoriatic patients, and evaluation of a psoriatic and arthritic questionnaire.** *J Rheumatol* 2002; 29:2577–2582.
2. Kane D, Stafford L, Bresnihan B *et al.* **A prospective, clinical and radiological study of early psoriatic arthritis: an early synovitis clinic experience.** *Rheumatology* 2003; 42:1460–1468.
3. Moll JM, Wright V. **Familial occurrence of psoriatic arthritis.** *Ann Rheum Dis* 1973; 32:181–201.
4. Stankler L. **An experimental investigation on the site of skin damage inducing the Koebner reaction in psoriasis.** *Br J Dermatol* 1969; 81: 534–535.
5. Rasmussen JE. **The relationship between infection with group A beta hemolytic streptococci and the development of psoriasis.** *Pediatr Infect Dis J* 2000; 19:153–154.
6. Rahman MU, Ahmed S, Schumacher HR *et al.* **High levels of antipeptidoglycan antibodies in psoriatic and other seronegative arthritides.** *J Rheumatol* 1990; 17:621–625.
7. Thomssen H, Hoffmann B, Schank M *et al.* **There is no disease-specific role for streptococci-responsive synovial T lymphocytes in the pathogenesis of psoriatic arthritis.** *Med Microbiol Immunol* 2000; 188:203–207.
8. Leung DY, Travers JB, Giorno R *et al.* **Evidence for a streptococcal superantigen-driven process in acute guttate psoriasis.** *J Clin Invest* 1995; 96: 2106–2112.
9. Ellis CN, Fradin MS, Messana JM *et al.* **Cyclosporine for plaque-type psoriasis. Results of a multidose, double-blind trial.** *N Engl J Med* 1991; 324: 277–284.
10. Wrone-Smith T, Nickoloff BJ. **Dermal injection of immunocytes induces psoriasis.** *J Clin Invest* 1996; 98:1878–1887.
11. Veale D, Yanni G, Rogers S *et al.* **Reduced synovial membrane macrophage numbers, ELAM-1 expression, and lining layer hyperplasia in psoriatic arthritis as compared with rheumatoid arthritis.** *Arthritis Rheum* 1993; 36:893–900.
12. Reece RJ, Canete JD, Parsons WJ *et al.* **Distinct vascular patterns of early synovitis in psoriatic, reactive, and rheumatoid arthritis.** *Arthritis Rheum* 1999; 42:1481–1484.
13. Fearon U, Griosios K, Fraser A *et al.* **Angiopoietins, growth factors, and vascular morphology in early arthritis.** *J Rheumatol* 2003; 30:260–268.
14. Ritchlin C, Haas-Smith SA, Hicks D *et al.* **Patterns of cytokine production in psoriatic synovium.** *J Rheumatol* 1998; 25:1544–1552.
15. Moll JM, Wright V. **Psoriatic arthritis.** *Semin Arthritis Rheum* 1973; 3:55–78.
16. McGonagle D, Gibbon W, O'Connor P *et al.* **Characteristic magnetic resonance imaging entheseal changes of knee synovitis in spondylarthropathy.** *Arthritis Rheum* 1998; 41:694–700.
17. Laloux L, Voisin MC, Allain J *et al.* **Immunohistological study of entheses in spondyloarthropathies: comparison in rheumatoid arthritis and osteoarthritis.** *Ann Rheum Dis* 2001; 60:316–321.
18. Marzo-Ortega H, McGonagle D, O'Connor P *et al.* **Efficacy of etanercept in the treatment of the entheseal pathology in resistant spondylarthropathy: a clinical and magnetic resonance imaging study.** *Arthritis Rheum* 2001; 44:2112–2117.
19. Ritchlin CT, Haas-Smith SA, Li P *et al.* **Mechanisms of TNF-alpha- and RANKL-mediated osteoclastogenesis and bone resorption in psoriatic arthritis.** *J Clin Invest* 2003; 111:821–831.
20. Suda T, Takahashi N, Udagawa N *et al.* **Modulation of osteoclast differentiation and function by the new members of the tumor necrosis factor receptor and ligand families.** *Endocr Rev* 1999; 20:345–357.
21. Lacey DL, Timms E, Tan HL *et al.* **Osteoprotegerin ligand is a cytokine that regulates osteoclast differentiation and activation.** *Cell* 1998; 93:165–176.
22. Hofbauer LC, Heufelder AE. **The role of osteoprotegerin and receptor activator of nuclear factor kappaB ligand in the pathogenesis and treatment of rheumatoid arthritis.** *Arthritis Rheum* 2001; 44:253–259.
23. Resnick D NG. **Psoriatic arthritis.** In: *Bone and Joint Imaging.* Edited by D Resnick. Philadelphia: WB Saunders, 1989; 320–329.
24. Peng H, Wright V, Usas A *et al.* **Synergistic enhancement of bone formation and healing by stem cell-expressed VEGF and bone morphogenetic protein-4.** *J Clin Invest* 2002; 110:751–759.
25. Austin LM, Ozawa M, Kikuchi T *et al.* **The majority of epidermal T cells in Psoriasis vulgaris lesions can produce type 1 cytokines, interferon-gamma, interleukin-2, and tumor necrosis factor-alpha, defining TC1 (cytotoxic T lymphocyte) and TH1 effector populations: a type 1 differentiation bias is also measured in circulating blood T cells in psoriatic patients.** *J Invest Dermatol* 1999; 113: 752–759.
26. Vervoordeldonk MJ, Tak PP. **Cytokines in rheumatoid arthritis.** *Curr Rheumatol Rep* 2002; 4:208–217.

27. Danning CL, Illei GG, Hitchon C *et al.* **Macrophage-derived cytokine and nuclear factor kappaB p65 expression in synovial membrane and skin of patients with psoriatic arthritis.** *Arthritis Rheum* 2000; **43**:1244–1256.

28. Ammora L, Jones A. **Unusual and memorable. Acro-osteolysis of the terminal phalanges.** *Ann Rheum Dis* 1998; **57**:389.

29. Ribbens C, Martin Y, Porras M, Franchimont N *et al.* **Increased matrix metalloproteinase-3 serum levels in rheumatic diseases: relationship with synovitis and steroid treatment.** *Ann Rheum Dis* 2002; **61**:161–166.

30. Vandooren B, Kruitof E, Yu DT *et al.* **Involvement of matrix metalloproteinases and their inhibitors in peripheral synovitis and down-regulation by tumor necrosis factor alpha blockade in spondylarthropathy.** *Arthritis Rheum* 2004; **50**: 2942–2953.

31. Vaz A, Barton J, Ritchlin C. **Psoriatic arthritis: an update for clinicians.** *Intl J Adv Rheumatol* 2005; **2**:126–134.

3
Clinical Evaluation

Philip Helliwell

Although psoriatic arthritis (PsA) was initially thought to be a variant of rheumatoid arthritis (RA), the pioneering work of Wright and Baker identified the distinctive features of the arthritis occurring in association with psoriasis [1]. Wright described the frequent involvement of distal interphalangeal (DIP) joints with erosion and absorption of the terminal phalanges and frequent reduction of bone stock in the other digits leading to a mutilating form of arthritis. Wright also described sacroiliitis and spondylitis occurring alone and in association with peripheral arthritis. The original five clinical subgroups described by Moll and Wright are still in use today, although the validity of this classification has been challenged [2].

Wright and Moll later defined the concept of the seronegative spondyloarthropathies (SpAs) as a group of disorders sharing common clinical features, including (as a hallmark feature) sacroiliitis, a seronegative (for rheumatoid factor) anodular asymmetric peripheral oligoarthritis, a hyperkeratotic and sometimes pustular rash on the hands and soles (keratoderma blenorrhagica), peripheral and central enthesitis, anterior uveitis, and familial aggregation [3]. The discovery of the high prevalence of human leukocyte antigen (HLA)-B27 in ankylosing spondylitis and other diseases in this group provided confirmation of this concept. PsA fit very well into the SpA group, often demonstrating many of the shared clinical features described above. It is therefore sometimes difficult to differentiate PsA from other SpAs, such as reactive arthritis and ankylosing spondylitis. Pure axial disease in association with psoriasis may resemble classic ankylosing spondylitis but it is usually less severe with atypical radiologic features.

Despite clinical, radiologic and familial evidence supporting PsA as a distinct disease entity, controversy still exists about which patients to include within this disease group. Some authors have even questioned whether PsA is a separate disease, suggesting that psoriasis merely modifies the expression of pre-existing RA. Other authors have argued that new onset chronic polyarthritis is undifferentiated and only evolves into a more distinctive form with time, such that the presence of psoriasis at onset of disease is of no value in nosologic terms [4]. The problem is not with the classic presentation of PsA – with oligoarthritis, DIP joint involvement, calcaneal enthesitis and dactylitis – but with the group of patients who have seronegative polyarthritis and psoriasis.

Overall, the sex ratio in PsA approximates unity but will vary across the subgroups so that males predominate in the spondylitis and oligoarthritis groups, while females predominate in the most frequent subgroup, symmetric polyarthritis, as also occurs in RA.

The peak age of onset of PsA is similar to that found in RA (20–40 years). In most cases, this is later than the onset of psoriasis so that the psoriasis precedes the arthritis in PsA. However, a potential source of diagnostic confusion occurs when the arthritis precedes the psoriasis, as it does in 15–20% of cases [5]. For this reason it is important for the physician to check thoroughly for clinical stigmata of psoriasis, including examination of the nails, scalp, the soles and palms, and the flexural areas, particularly the natal cleft.

Clinical evaluation of patients with suspected PsA should be systematic and include an assessment of the skin, the entheses, and the spine. The importance of family history cannot be overemphasized as part of the clinical evaluation because of familial clustering, initially described by Wright and others. Evaluation of the established case should include an assessment of the skin and joints, taking into account the distinctive features of PsA. Although there are well-established ways of measuring the skin involvement, many clinicians make a quasi-objective appraisal and record

'mild, moderate, or severe'. From the articular point of view, evaluation involves performing a 78 tender joint/76 swollen joint count to include the DIP joints, assessing the presence of dactylitis and enthesitis and the severity of spinal involvement, if relevant.

In the clinic situation it often helps to have a *pro forma* to aid this complex assessment process and to facilitate recording of data. Radiologic studies can help clarify the diagnosis with a minimum plain radiographic set of hands, feet, and pelvis. The frequency of asymptomatic sacroiliitis in PsA should prompt the physician to X-ray these joints if there is diagnostic suspicion of PsA. In early disease, when plain radiographs are normal, magnetic resonance imaging (MRI) can be of help as MRI changes precede plain radiographic abnormalities (*see* Chapter 4, *Imaging*).

PsA clinical subgroups of Moll and Wright

Distal interphalangeal predominant disease (5%)

Asymmetric oligoarthritis (70%)

Symmetric polyarthritis (15%)

Predominant spinal involvement (5%)

Arthritis mutilans (5%)

Figure 3.1. Clinical subgroups of Moll and Wright are shown, with their respective percent contribution to the whole group [6]. Although this classification is still widely used, other classifications have been proposed, largely to simplify and provide a basis for explanatory studies [2,7]. However, it is clear that the proportion of each of the original Moll and Wright subgroups has changed with recent publications, the symmetric polyarthritis subgroup now being the predominant group. Assuming that there have been no fundamental changes to the disease in the last 40 years, it must be concluded that subsequent authors have identified cases in a different way than Moll and Wright. The original criteria were designed to be sensitive without being too specific, but it is likely that Moll and Wright were using other features of the disease to make their diagnosis. In other words they were using implicit, but undeclared, features to enhance the specificity of their criteria. Later authors, unaware of this, have interpreted the Moll and Wright criteria to the latter – resulting in the inclusion of more patients with symmetric polyarthritis. As a result of this, it is possible that some of the patients included in the later series have seronegative rheumatoid arthritis (RA) with coincidental psoriasis.

DIP joint inflammation

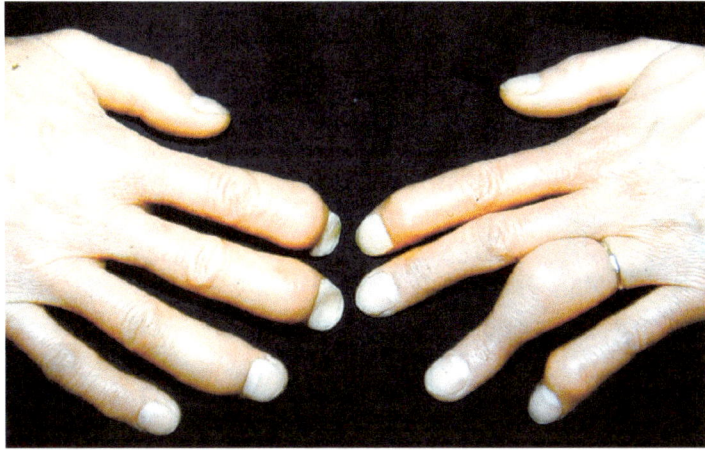

FIGURE 3.2. Distal interphalangeal (DIP) joint inflammation is a hallmark of this disease and is frequently seen in association with psoriasis of the nails. Involvement of the DIP joint in psoriatic arthritis (PsA) is almost always associated with psoriatic nail changes. Despite this, isolated DIP joint involvement in PsA may be missed, even by experienced observers [8]. Psoriatic onychopathy may be linked independently to inflammatory and osteolytic changes in the distal phalanx, even in the absence of PsA. In the absence of psoriasis, clinical involvement of the DIP joints may be indistinguishable from inflammatory osteoarthritis. However, DIP inflammation may present in such a way as to leave no doubt about the diagnosis with characteristic involvement of the interphalangeal joints of the thumb and great toes (the eponymous Bauer's digit) and of the DIP joints of the feet, rarely described in osteoarthritis. If there is doubt clinically, radiologic studies should help to separate inflammatory osteoarthritis from PsA as the latter, apart from producing characteristic differences at the joint ('whiskering' due to juxta-articular new bone formation), may also produce typical changes in the terminal phalanx, including tuft erosion and osteolysis [9].

Asymmetric oligoarthritis

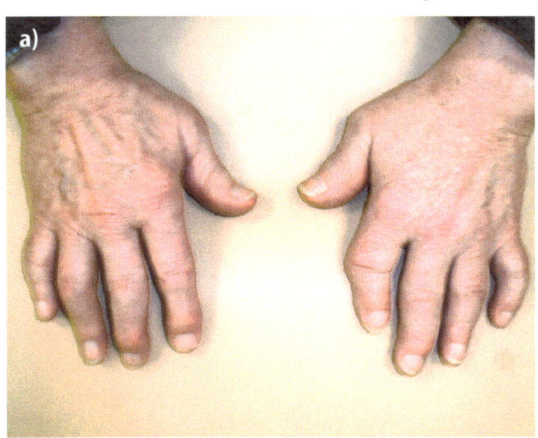
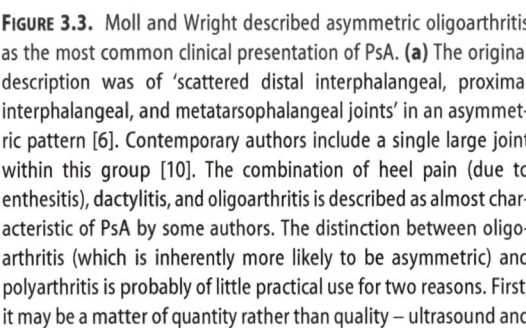
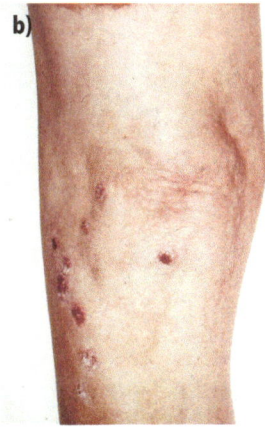
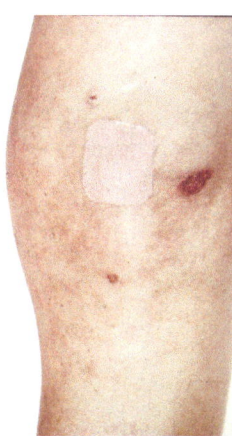

FIGURE 3.3. Moll and Wright described asymmetric oligoarthritis as the most common clinical presentation of PsA. **(a)** The original description was of 'scattered distal interphalangeal, proximal interphalangeal, and metatarsophalangeal joints' in an asymmetric pattern [6]. Contemporary authors include a single large joint within this group [10]. The combination of heel pain (due to enthesitis), dactylitis, and oligoarthritis is described as almost characteristic of PsA by some authors. The distinction between oligoarthritis (which is inherently more likely to be asymmetric) and polyarthritis is probably of little practical use for two reasons. First, it may be a matter of quantity rather than quality – ultrasound and magnetic resonance imaging (MRI) have demonstrated subclinical involvement of joints and an outward oligoarthritis may in fact be a polyarthritis if non-involved joints are examined by these imaging techniques. Second, joint patterns evolve with time, most commonly from an oligoarthritis at presentation to a polyarthritis as time passes [11]. **(b)** Nevertheless, the patient with a persistently swollen knee who experiences recurrent massive effusions but with minimal pain and disability is sometimes seen in this condition and probably does not progress as would be expected for other inflammatory arthritides. Part **(b)** reproduced with permission from [10].

Symmetric polyarthritis

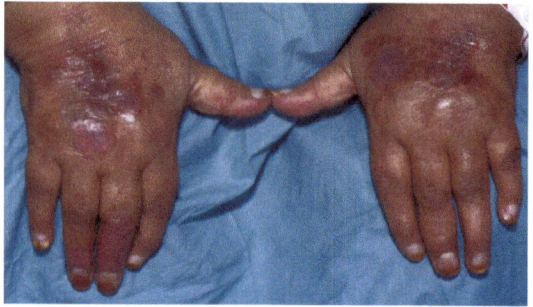

FIGURE 3.4. Although comprising only 15% of the original cohort described by Moll and Wright, an increasing proportion of patients are now described with symmetric polyarthritis. Clinically, the arthritis may resemble RA. The distinction between RA and PsA is sometimes difficult to make clinically, particularly in the face of psoriasis and a negative rheumatoid factor. It is helpful to look for other distinguishing features such as DIP involvement, enthesopathy, dactylitis, and axial involvement. Conversely, the presence of rheumatoid nodules and systemic features of disease would favor RA. Other serologic tests may help: anti-cyclic citrullinated peptide antibodies are highly specific for RA.

Classic ankylosing spondylitis

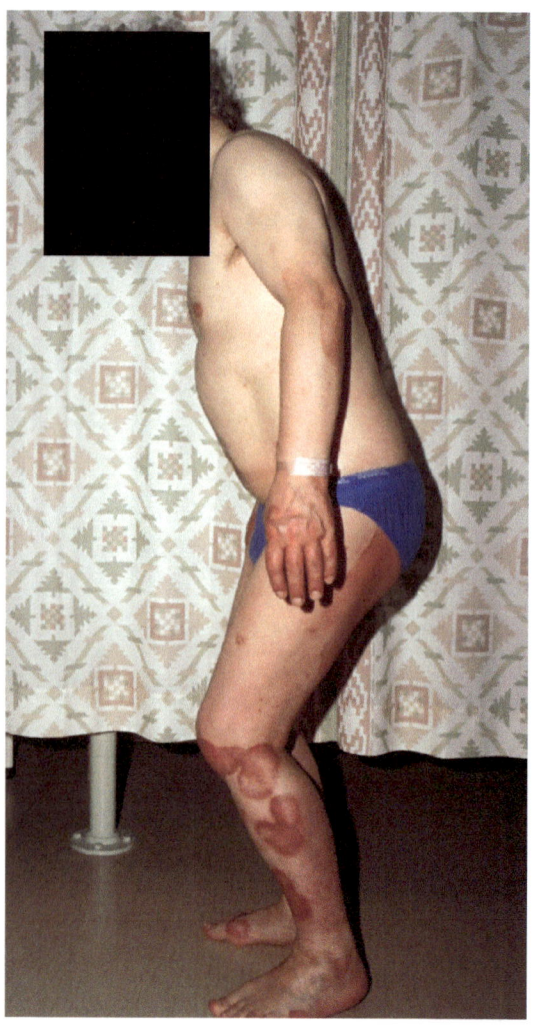

FIGURE 3.5. Although classic ankylosing spondylitis is seen in association with psoriasis, radiographic differences between classic ankylosing spondylitis (and the spondylitis associated with inflammatory bowel disease) and psoriatic spondylitis (and the spondylitis associated with reactive arthritis) suggest a different phenotype. Further, axial radiographic changes may occur in PsA in the absence of symptoms. It is perhaps more compelling to regard the issue as one of quantity rather than quality – the disease is merely less extensive in PsA rather than a completely different disease process. The radiographic differences can be summarized as: asymmetric sacroiliitis; more frequent non-marginal 'chunky' syndesmophytes; less frequent marginal syndesmophytes; paravertebral ossification; and more frequent involvement of cervical spine. The prevalence of spondylitis depends, to some extent, on the method used to identify spinal involvement. Clinical maneuvers to test sacroiliac joint involvement are generally thought to be insensitive. Williamson *et al.* [12] have demonstrated poor sensitivity (38%) and specificity (67%) of clinical tests for sacroiliac involvement. Clearly, diagnosis and classification on symptoms alone are insufficient and some form of objective imaging appears necessary to complete the picture. The cost and limited availability of MRI make plain radiography more attractive for the purpose of classification, although MRI seems more sensitive for detecting early disease.

Distinctive mutilation in PsA

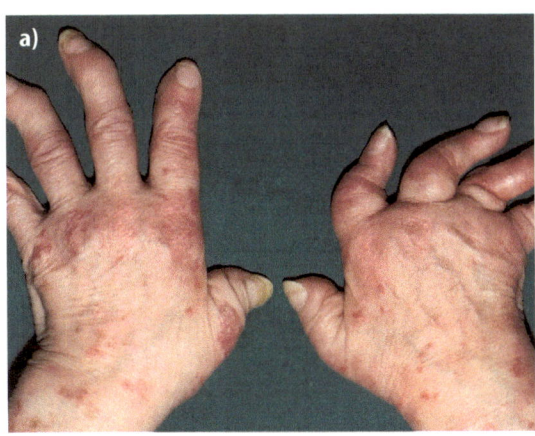

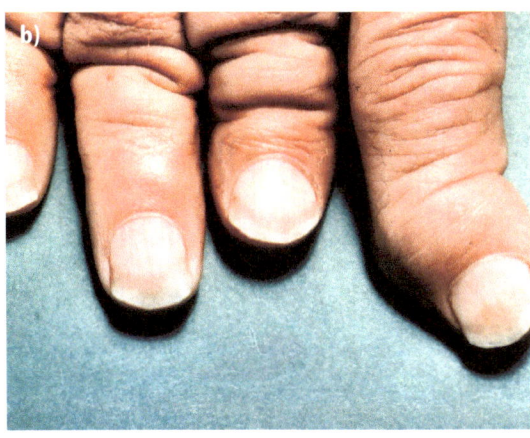

FIGURE 3.6. Although a mutilating form of arthritis can be seen in RA, a distinctive form of mutilation is seen very occasionally in PsA **(a,b)**. This severe mutilating arthritis is characterized by widespread digital deformity and the presence of flail digits with redundant folds of skin. Radiographically extensive phalangeal osteolysis is seen, sometimes coexisting with joint ankylosis in the same digits. As the condition is seldom seen, it has been impossible to predict who will develop such deformities at disease onset, unless, of course, such changes are present at presentation.

Dactylitis in the hand and foot

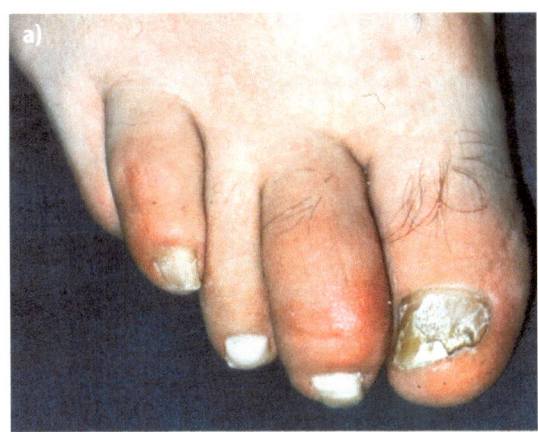

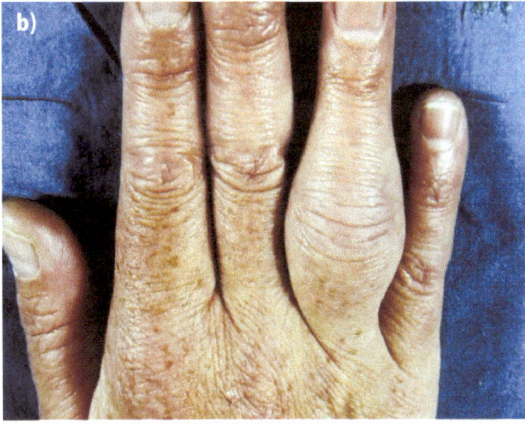

FIGURE 3.7. Dactylitis is one of the hallmark clinical features of PsA occurring in 16–48% of reported cases [2,5]. **(a,b)** Dactylitis is characterized by uniform swelling of the digit. According to some authors, dactylitis is predominantly due to swelling and inflammation in the flexor tendon sheaths [13], although other groups have recorded joint synovitis as well as tenosynovitis [14]. Chronic, non-tender, diffuse dactylitic swelling occurs in PsA and may be less of an indicator of active disease than tenderness within the swollen digit. Rarely, unilateral limb edema is seen in PsA and, although there are clinical similarities with the limb edema seen in RA (where an abnormality of lymphatic vessels has been described), this may be an extreme example of 'limb dactylitis' (*see* Figure 3.12).

Entheseal sites in PsA

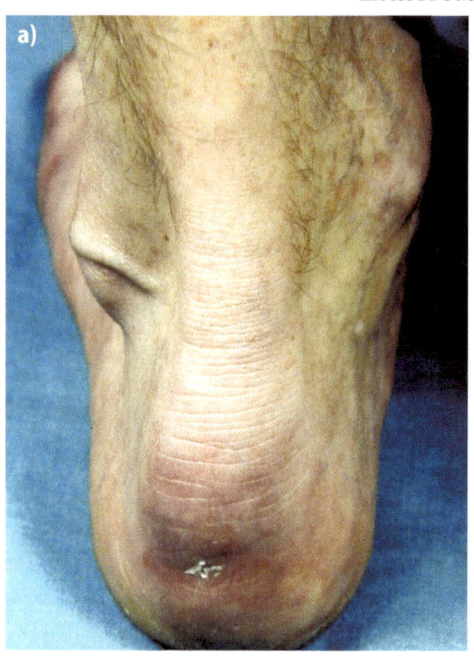 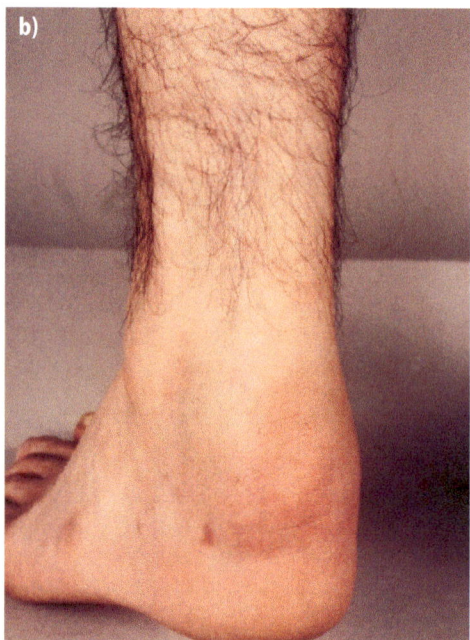

FIGURE 3.8. McGonagle *et al.* [15] rekindled interest in the enthesis as the major site of pathology underlying PsA. There are literally hundreds of entheseal sites (sites of attachment of ligament and tendon to bone). The most common sites involved in PsA are the calcaneum (both at the attachment of the Achilles tendon **[a,b]** and at the attachment of the plantar fascia), at muscular and tendon attachments around the pelvis, the inferior aspect of the patella, and the elbow. Tenderness at these specific sites is sufficient to diagnose involvement, and sometimes swelling is obvious at the tendinous or ligamentous insertion. Spondylitis may in fact be regarded as an example of multiple sites of enthesitis with syndesmophytes representing bony 'spurs'. The specificity of enthesitis in PsA remains to be determined as an ultrasonographic study of calcaneal enthesitis demonstrated bony erosion at the enthesis more often in RA than in PsA [16].

SAPHO syndrome – palmoplantar pustulosis

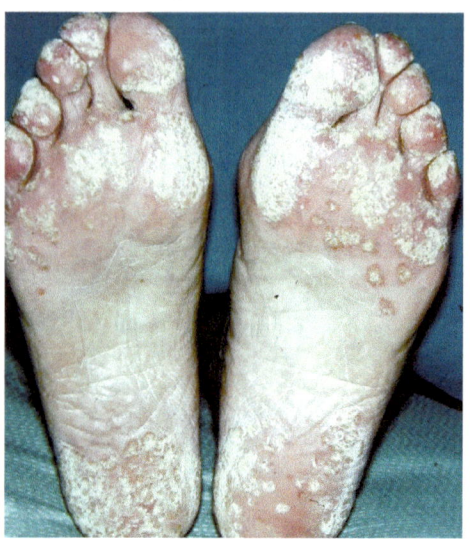

FIGURE 3.9. Palmoplantar pustulosis and other pustular conditions, such as acne conglobata, acne fulminans, and hidradenitis suppurativa, are associated with a distinct collection of osteoarticular associations, including sternoclavicular hyperostosis, chronic sterile recurrent multifocal osteomyelitis, hyperostosis of the spine, and, occasionally, a peripheral arthritis. These associated clinical features have been grouped together as the synovitis, acne, pustulosis, hyperostosis, and osteomyelitis (SAPHO) syndrome. The condition seems to be common in Japan [17] but it has been described worldwide, with French authors foremost [18].

SAPHO syndrome – abnormal radioisotope uptake in psoriasis vulgaris

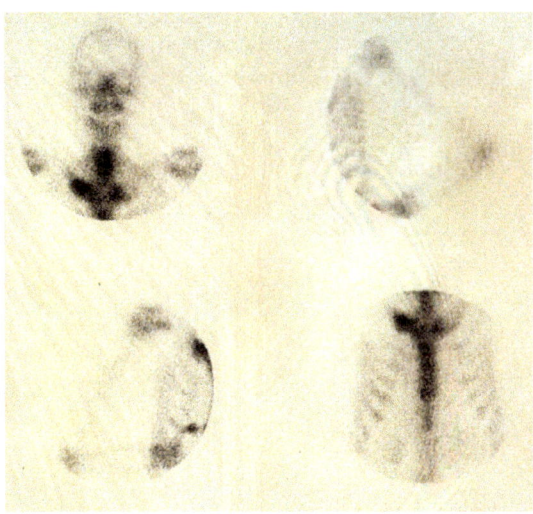

FIGURE 3.10. Further studies have shown abnormal uptake of radioisotope in the manubriosternal and sternoclavicular joints in association with psoriasis vulgaris in patients already given a diagnosis of PsA. This suggests that SAPHO syndrome should be included within the spectrum of PsA [2].

Eye disease in PsA

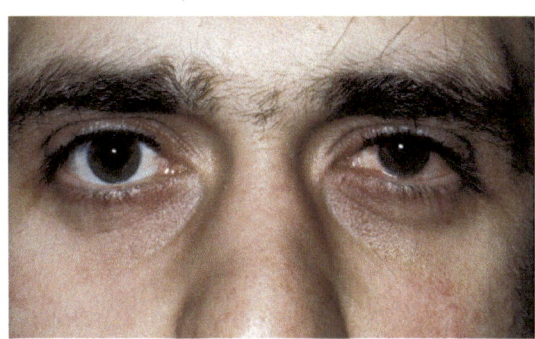

FIGURE 3.11. Eye disease is commonly seen in PsA. In an unselected series of 112 patients ocular inflammation was reported in almost one-third, although most of these cases had conjunctival inflammation [19]. Uveitis was found in 7%. Other series have suggested a higher prevalence of uveitis (18%), but it is generally agreed that uveitis is less common in PsA than in ankylosing spondylitis, possibly reflecting the lower frequency of axial involvement in PsA. Two forms of uveitis are recognized: acute anterior uveitis, similar to that found in ankylosing spondylitis, and an uveitis of more insidious onset, which is frequently a bilateral, chronic anterior and posterior disease associated with human leukocyte antigen (HLA)-DR13 rather than HLA-B27 [20].

Pitting edema in PsA

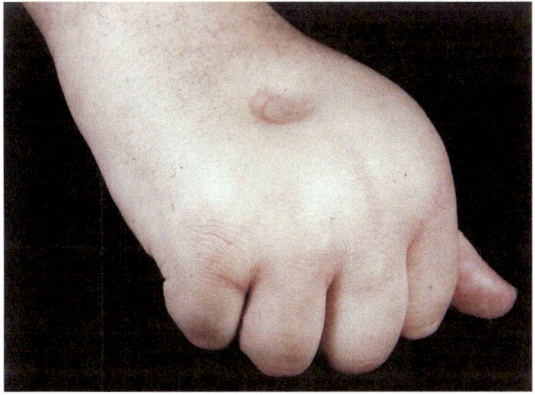

FIGURE 3.12. Pitting edema of one or both upper limbs has been described in association with PsA. Since so few cases have been described, it is difficult to make firm associations. Mulherin *et al.* [21] described four cases and concluded that the edema was unrelated to the extent or severity of the arthritis. Lymphoscintigraphy showed delayed clearance of the isotope, similar to that seen with limb edema in RA. The edema is usually refractory to treatment but may respond to disease-modifying anti-rheumatic therapy. Supportive measures such as compression hosiery are recommended.

Relationship between joint symmetry and number of joints in PsA

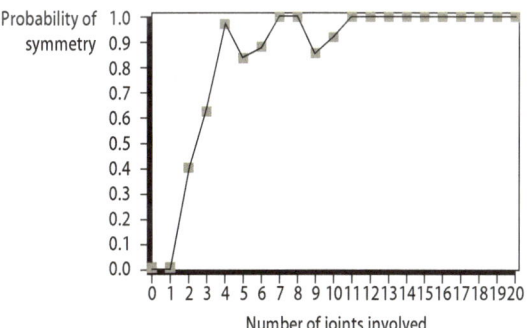

FIGURE 3.13. This graph shows the relationship between joint symmetry (defined as more than 50% of joints occurring as matched pairs) and the number of joints involved. The data were obtained from 77 patients with PsA (29 women and 48 men). Their mean age was 53 years and the mean duration of disease was 14 years. The probability of having symmetric disease is given on the vertical axis: the greater the number of joints involved, the more likely symmetric disease is present. When more than 12 joints are involved, symmetry is obligatory. PsA is usually described as being less symmetric than RA. However, as indicated above, this is purely a reflection of the number of joints involved clinically. The fact that early and late PsA have fewer joints involved than RA accounts for the asymmetry described in this disease.

Juvenile PsA

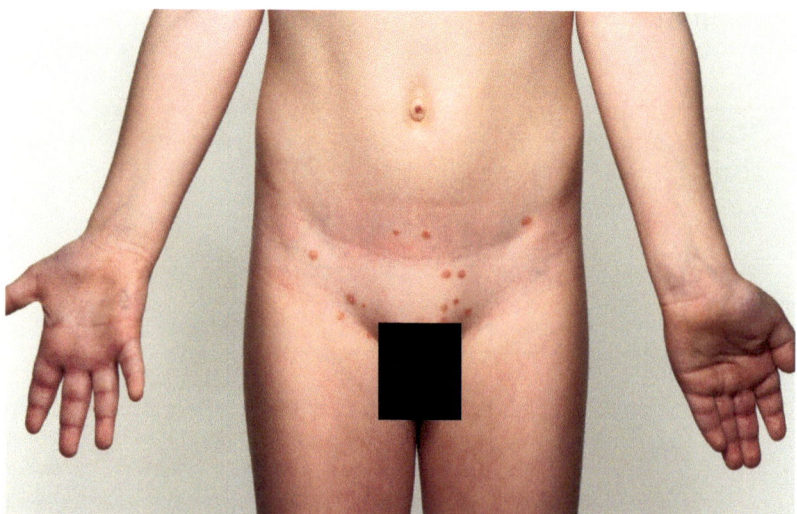

FIGURE 3.14. Juvenile PsA is uncommon. Unlike adult PsA, arthritis often precedes psoriasis (52% of cases). The commonest clinical findings in children are an asymmetric polyarthritis often involving the digits. Patients may also present with a single swollen joint (such as a knee) and with spondylitis. Both dactylitis and eye involvement may occur, the latter in association with a positive antinuclear factor, as may be seen in other cases of juvenile idio-pathic arthritis (JIA). Classification criteria for juvenile arthritis continue to evolve [22]. The Durban criteria require the presence of arthritis and psoriasis *or* arthritis and at least two of dactylitis, nail abnormalities consistent with psoriasis, and a family history of psoriasis. The first two criteria are likely to be sensitive but not specific for juvenile PsA. The second three criteria recognize that arthritis may occur in the absence of psoriasis in this group.

HIV and PsA

Compatible clinical profile

- Severe widespread psoriaform lesions with onychopathy occurring *de novo* in an adult at risk of HIV disease

- Male predominance

- Severe enthesitis, usually calcaneal

- Aggressive large joint lower limb oligoarthritis

Laboratory investigations

- Rheumatoid factor and antinuclear factor usually negative

- Reduced CD4 T-lymphocyte count

- Widespread entheseal inflammation on MRI scan

FIGURE 3.15. In the 1980s, reports suggested a link between psoriasis and HIV infection, of interest being the extensive skin disease associated with AIDS, including widespread confluent patches and severe onychodystrophy. Subsequently, the association between HIV, AIDS, severe psoriasis, and the spondyloarthropathies (SpAs) has been confirmed in African countries where SpA was virtually unknown prior to the outbreak of HIV/AIDS [23]. The association has provided some insights into the pathogenesis of the disease and has emphasized the importance of the CD8 lymphocyte in both the skin and the joint disorder [24]. Distinctive features of the arthropathy associated with HIV include severe enthesitis (particularly about the heel), dactylitis, and rapidly progressive, lower limb joint destruction. Axial involvement is seen less frequently. Under these circumstances, it may be difficult to distinguish cases of PsA from reactive arthritis, or even septic arthritis, as many of these patients are immunocompromised and may have unusual infections.

Clinical syndromes that suggest PsA

- Monoarthritis, usually of knee joint, often with huge effusion but little disability or pain

- Oligoarthritis of scattered PIP and DIP joints of hands and feet

- Pain and swelling of first interphalangeal joint of great toe with enthesitis of heel and a dactylitic toe

- Polyarthritis of large and small joints including DIP joints

FIGURE 3.16. PsA may present in one of several ways. The key features of the classical presentation are summarized in this figure. The main difficulty is differentiation from other common forms of arthritis at presentation. PIP, proximal interphalangeal.

General diagnostic principles for PsA

Compatible clinical profile

- No gender preference (males:females)
- Age of onset 20–40 years
- Racial preference
- Usual clinical evidence of psoriasis (but arthritis precedes psoriasis in 15–20% cases)
- Frequently oligoarticular at disease onset

Laboratory investigations

- Rheumatoid factor and antinuclear factor usually negative
- CRP may be normal and less helpful in monitoring activity of disease
- HLA analysis not usually helpful in diagnosis

FIGURE 3.17. Overall, the sex ratio in PsA approximates unity but will vary across the subgroups so that male predominance occurs in the spondylitis predominant form, while females predominate in the most frequent subgroup – symmetrical polyarthritis. Racial differences in the prevalence of psoriasis are reflected in the prevalence of PsA, although precise epidemiology of PsA across ethnic groups is lacking, partly because of a lack of agreed classification criteria. The peak age of onset of PsA is similar to that found in RA (20–40 years). This is, in most cases, later than the onset of psoriasis, which appears for the most part between 5 and 15 years of age. This is reflected by the figures for onset of arthritis and psoriasis; psoriasis precedes arthritis in the majority of cases. However, a potential source of diagnostic confusion occurs when arthritis precedes psoriasis as it does in 15–20% of cases.

In a minority of cases PsA may also be first diagnosed at the extremes of life. The most recent criteria for classifying JIA include a specific subgroup for PsA yet use psoriasis as an exclusion for the group labeled 'enthesitis-related arthritis' (*see* Figure 3.14). Additionally, there has been some interest in elderly onset PsA, which appears to differ only slightly from classical PsA, the most notable difference being the lower prevalence of spinal disease in this cohort. There are no biological markers for this condition. A negative test for rheumatoid factor is reassuring but not mandatory. A positive test for antibodies to citrullinated proteins makes the diagnosis of PsA less likely. Conventional radiology at onset is seldom useful but other modalities such as MRI may have a place, although the sensitivity and specificity of, for example, MRI evidence of enthesitis is unknown. Occasionally there may be evidence of bilateral sacroiliitis at onset of peripheral joint disease. CRP, C-reactive protein.

Flexural psoriasis

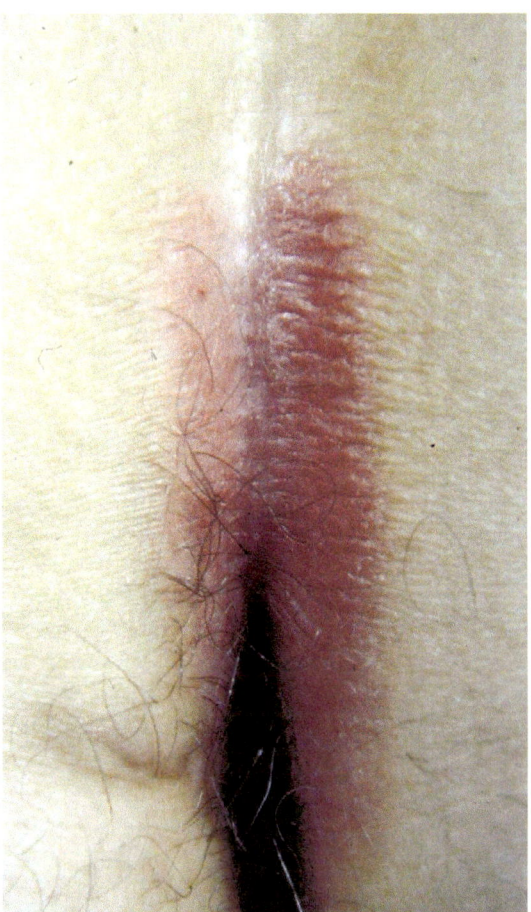

FIGURE 3.18. A 37-year-old fit and active male presented with a history of recurrent massive swelling of both knees over a period of 11 years. He had had repeated drainage and injection of corticosteroids but had been able to continue running between episodes. Rheumatoid factor was negative. Examination revealed grossly swollen knees and a patch of flexural psoriasis in his natal cleft. Radiology revealed unilateral sacroiliitis. He responded well to radiosynovectomy with yttrium-90.

Left and right hand of a 67-year-old male at first presentation

a)

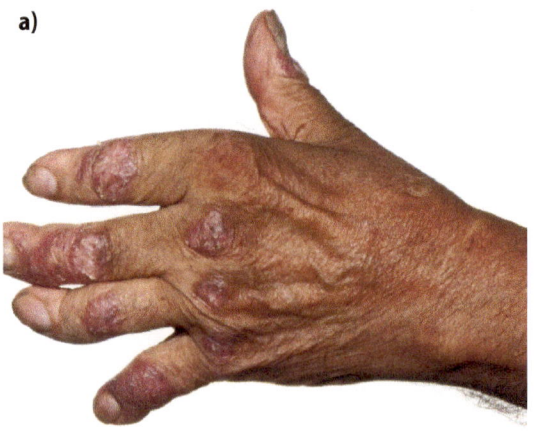

b)

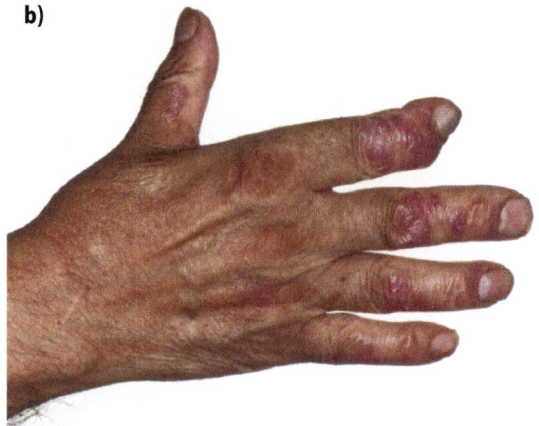

FIGURE 3.19. At this time he had been visiting his primary care physician for 9 years with 'rheumatoid arthritis'. He had pain and stiffness in his left shoulder, left hand, and knees. He said that he had had psoriasis for 26 years. Examination revealed osteoarthritis of his knees. He had synovitis of the second and third left metacar- pophalangeal joints, left wrist, and dactylitis of his left index finger **(a)** with deformity of his right index **(b)** and left middle DIP joints. Radiographs showed osteolysis of the left second toe terminal phalanx and normal sacroiliac joints.

Inflammatory articular disease (joint, spine, or entheseal)

With 3 or more points from the following:

1. Evidence of psoriasis (one of a, b, c)	(a) Current psoriasis*	*Psoriatic skin or scalp disease present today as judged by a rheumatologist or dermatologist*
	(b) Personal history of psoriasis	*A history of psoriasis that may be obtained from patient, family doctor, dermatologist, rheumatologist or other qualified health-care provider*
	(c) Family history of psoriasis	*A history of psoriasis in a first or second degree relative according to patient report*
2. Psoriatic nail dystrophy		*Typical psoriatic nail dystrophy including onycholysis, pitting and hyperkeratosis observed on current physical examination*
3. A negative test for rheumatoid factor		*By any method except latex but preferably by ELISA or nephelometry, according to the local laboratory reference range*
4. Dactylitis (one of a, b)	(a) Current	*Swelling of an entire digit*
	(b) History	*A history of dactylitis recorded by a rheumatologist*
5. Radiological evidence of juxta-articular new bone formation		*Ill-defined ossification near joint margins (but excluding osteophyte formation) on plain xrays of hand or foot*

Specificity 0.987, sensitivity 0.914

*Current psoriasis scores 2 whereas all other items score 1

FIGURE 3.21. Dermatologists and other specialists wishing to ask specific questions to screen for PsA should use the adjacent list. The list is derived from a validated, self-administered tool used to screen patients with psoriasis for PsA [30]. A score of 4 was found to have a sensitivity of 60% and a specificity of 62%. However, just a combination of positive answers to questions 1 and 4a had a sensitivity of 30% and a specificity of 91% for axial and peripheral disease.

Screening questions for arthritis

Question	Score if positive
1. Have you ever thought you might have arthritis?	1
2. Have you ever had a swollen joint (or joints)?	2
3. Has a doctor ever told you that you have arthritis?	0
4. Are your joints stiff when you wake up in the morning?	1
4a. If yes, how long does the stiffness last?	1 if >60 mins
5. Have you ever had back trouble ?	0
6. Has your back ever been stiff in the morning?	0
6a. If yes, how long does the stiffness last?	1 if >60 mins
7. Do your nails have holes or pits?	
8. Do your fingernails come loose from the nail bed?	1 for any two positive responses: maximum score 2
9. Are your nails abnormally thick?	
10. Does anyone in your family have arthritis?	0

FIGURE 3.20. The CASPAR classification criteria for psoriatic arthritis. The CASPAR study group was established to derive new data driven classification criteria for psoriatic arthritis. Data were collected in 32 centres world wide by people with acknowledged expertise in this condition. Altogether over 100 clinical, radiological and laboratory variables were collected. The new criteria were derived by logistic regression and CART analysis (as a cross check). The CASPAR criteria gratifyingly have both characteristic dermatological, clinical and radiological features and have both high sensitivity and very high specificity (31). For traditionalists it is important to note that the Moll and Wright criteria (arthritis, psoriasis and negative rheumatoid factor), used in most studies since 1973, are contained nicely within this new set. It is also interesting to note that, with these criteria, it is now possible to be rheumatoid factor positive and still be classified as having psoriatic arthritis, providing other characteristic features are present. Recent work suggests that these classification criteria function equally well as diagnostic criteria and, additionally, that they are useful in diagnosing early disease (32, 33). It is also worth noting that 13% of the 'controls' had ankylosing spondylitis so the statistical analyses were influenced **against** selecting spinal features as characteristic of psoriatic arthritis. If the controls had only consisted of rheumatoid arthritis cases then it is possible that specific spinal features may have appeared in the final criteria set. A more complete discussion of the new criteria is given in Helliwell (34).

Diagnostic pointers to distinguish PsA from RA

Favors PsA	Favors RA
Asymmetric oligoarticular	Symmetric polyarticular
Seronegative for rheumatoid factor and anti-CCP	Seropositive for rheumatoid factor and anti-CCP
Absence of rheumatoid nodules	Rheumatoid nodules over bony prominences
Dactylitis	
Enthesitis (heel, tibial apophysis)	
Psoriasis (scalp, plaque, guttate, flexural, nails) or family history of psoriasis	
DIP joint involvement	Features of systemic disease (cardiopulmonary involvement, vasculitis)
Uveitis	Episcleritis, scleritis
Clinical signs of sacroiliitis and spondylitis	
Plain radiograph: tuft osteolysis, DIP erosions, juxta-articular new bone formation, relative preservation of bone density, osteolysis, ankylosis of digital joints, entheseal new bone and erosion at entheseal insertion	Plain radiograph: marginal erosions, peri-articular osteoporosis, sparing of DIP joints
Axial radiography: sacroiliitis, spondylitis, paravertebral ossification	Axial radiography: facet joint destruction, occasional discitis, osteoporotic wedge fractures

FIGURE 3.22. Useful diagnostic pointers to distinguish PsA from RA. Seronegative symmetric polyarthritis with psoriasis may prove difficult to place from a taxonomic point of view. The above table may help in distinguishing PsA from RA in such cases. CCP, cyclic citrullinated peptide.

Distinguishing PsA from other SpAs

PsA	Reactive arthritis
Classic psoriatic plaques including scalp and flexural changes	Keratoderma blenorrhagica
	Circinate balanitis
Large and small joint arthritis including DIP joints	Predominant lower limb large joint arthritis
Uveitis	Conjunctivitis
Dactylitis may occur in both	
Enthesitis may occur in both	
Sacroiliitis may occur in both	

PsA	Ankylosing spondylitis
Psoriasis (scalp, plaque, guttate, flexural, nails) or family history of psoriasis	
Peripheral arthritis: large and small joint arthritis including DIP joints	Peripheral arthritis: predominant lower limb, large joint arthritis
Axial involvement may be asymptomatic	
Axial radiography:	Axial radiography:
• asymmetric sacroiliitis	• symmetric sacroiliitis
• paravertebral ossification	• marginal syndesmophytes
• non-marginal syndesmophytes	• symmetric syndesmophytes
• asymmetric syndesmophytes	• lumbar > cervical
• cervical > lumbar	• 'bamboo' spine

FIGURE 3.23. Classic ankylosing spondylitis may occur in association with psoriasis but distinct features of psoriatic spondylitis have been described (*see* Figure 3.5). A case of reactive arthritis where no infective trigger can be identified may be indistinguishable initially from PsA. Inflammatory bowel disease can also present with an asymmetric peripheral oligoarthritis prior to diagnosis of the bowel disorder – if a family history of psoriasis is also present then a misdiagnosis of PsA may be made.

References

1. Wright V. **Psoriatic arthritis: a comparative study of rheumatoid arthritis and arthritis associated with psoriasis.** *Ann Rheum Dis* 1961; 20:123.

2. Helliwell P, Marchesoni A, Peters M *et al.* **A re-evaluation of the osteoarticular manifestations of psoriasis.** *Br J Rheumatol* 1991; 30:339–345.

3. Wright V, Moll JMH. *Seronegative Polyarthritis.* Amsterdam: North Holland Publishing Co., 1976.

4. Harrison BJ, Silman AJ, Barrett EM *et al.* **Presence of psoriasis does not influence the presentation or short-term outcome of patients with early inflammatory polyarthritis.** *J Rheumatol* 1997; 24:1744–1749.

5. Gladman DD, Shuckett R, Russell ML *et al.* **Psoriatic arthritis (PSA) - an analysis of 220 patients.** *Quart J Med* 1987; 238:127–141.

6. Moll JMH, Wright V. **Psoriatic arthritis.** *Semin Arthritis Rheum* 1973; 3:51–78.

7. Veale D, Fitzgerald O. **Psoriatic arthritis – "DIP or not DIP? That is the question".** *Br J Rheumatol* 1992; 31:430–431.

8. Gorter S, van der Heijde DMFM, van der Linden S *et al.* **Psoriatic arthritis: performance of rheumatologists in daily practice.** *Ann Rheum Dis* 2002; 61:219–224.

9. Avila R, Pugh DG, Slocumb CH *et al.* **Psoriatic arthritis: a roentgenological study.** *Radiology* 1960; 75:691.

10. Helliwell PS, Wight V. **Psoriatic arthritis: clinical features.** In: *Rheumatology.* Edited by JH Klippel, PA Dieppe. London: Mosby; 1998; 6.21.1–6.21.8.

11. Jones SM, Armas JB, Cohen MG *et al.* **Psoriatic arthritis: outcome of disease subsets and relationship of joint disease to nail and skin disease.** *Br J Rheumatol* 1994; 33:834–839.

12. Williamson L, Dockerty JL, Dalbeth N *et al.* **Clinical assessment of sacroiliitis and HLA-B27 are poor predictors of sacroiliitis diagnosed by magnetic**

resonance imaging in psoriatic arthritis. *Rheumatology* 2004; **43**:85–88.

13. Olivieri I, Barozzi L, Favaro L *et al.* **Dactylitis in patients with seronegative spondylarthropathy. Assessment by ultrasonography and magnetic resonance imaging.** *Arthritis Rheum* 1996; **39**:1524–1528.

14. Kane D, Greaney T, Bresnihan B *et al.* **Ultrasonography in the diagnosis and management of psoriatic dactylitis.** *J Rheumatol* 1999; **26**:1746–1751.

15. McGonagle D, Gibbon W, Emery P. **Classification of inflammatory arthritis by enthesitis.** *Lancet* 1998; **352**:1137–1140.

16. Falsetti P, Frediani B, Fioravanti A *et al.* **Sonographic study of calcaneal entheses in erosive osteoarthritis, nodal osteoarthritis, rheumatoid arthritis and psoriatic arthritis.** *Scand J Rheumatol* 2003; **32**:229–234.

17. Sonozaki H, Mitsui H, Miyanaga Y *et al.* **Clinical features of 53 cases with pustulotic arthro-osteitis.** *Ann Rheum Dis* 1981; **40**:547–553.

18. Benhamou C-L, Chamot AM, Kahn MF. **Synovitis-acnepustulosis hyperostosis-osteomyelitis syndrome (Sapho). A new syndrome among the spondyloarthropathies?** *Clin Exp Rheumatol* 1988; **6**:109–112.

19. Lambert JR, Wright V. **Eye inflammation in psoriatic arthritis.** *Ann Rheum Dis* 1976; **35**:354–356.

20. Queiro R, Torre JC, Belzunegui J *et al.* **Clinical features and predictive factors in psoriatic arthritis-related uveitis.** *Semin Arthritis Rheum* 2002; **31**:264–270.

21. Mulherin DM, Fitzgerald O, Bresnihan B. **Lymphedema of the upper limb in patients with psoriatic arthritis.** *Semin Arthritis Rheum* 1993; **22**:350–356.

22. Petty RE, Southwood TR, Baum J *et al.* **Revision of the proposed classification for juvenile idiopathic arthritis: Durban 1997.** *J Rheumatol* 1998; **25**:1991–1994.

23. Njobvu P, McGill P, Kerr H *et al.* **Spondyloarthropathy and HIV infection in Zambia.** *J Rheumatol* 1998; **25**:1553–1559.

24. Hohler T, Marker-Hermann E. **Psoriatic arthritis: clinical aspects, genetics, and the role of T cells.** *Curr Opin Rheumatol* 2001; **13**:273–279.

25. Bennett RM. **Psoriatic arthritis.** In: *Arthritis and Related Conditions.* DJ McCarty, ed. Philadelphia: Lea and Febiger; 1979; 645.

26. Taylor WJ, Marchesoni A, Arreghini M *et al.* **A comparison of the performance characteristics of classification criteria for the diagnosis of psoriatic arthritis.** *Semin Arthritis Rheum* 2004; **34**:575–584.

27. Vasey FB, Espinoza LR. **Psoriatic arthritis.** In: *Spondyloarthropathies.* Edited A Calin. Orlando: Grune and Stratton, 1987; 151–185.

28. Dougados M, van der Linden S, Juhlin R *et al.* **The European Spondyloarthropathy Study Group preliminary criteria for the classification of spondyloarthropathy.** *Arthritis Rheum* 1991; **34**:1218.

29. Fournie B, Crognier L, Arnaud C *et al.* **Proposed classification criteria of psoriatic arthritis: a preliminary study in 260 patients.** *Rev Rhum* (Engl edn) 1999; **66**:446–456.

30. Alenius GM, Stenberg B, Stenlund H *et al.* **Inflammatory joint manifestations are prevalent in psoriasis: prevalence study of joint and axial involvement in psoriatic patients, and evaluation of a psoriatic and arthritic questionnaire.** *J Rheumatol* 2002; **29**:2577–2582.

31. Taylor WJ, Gladman DD, Helliwell PS, Marchesoni A, Mease P, Mielants H et al. **Classification criteria for psoriatic arthritis: Development of new criteria from a large international study.** *Arthritis and Rheumatism* 2006; **54**(8):2665–2673.

32. Chandran V, Schentag C, Gladman DD. **CASPAR criteria are sensitive in early psoriatic arthritis.** *Arthritis and Rheumatism* **54**[Abstracts supplement], s794.

33. Chandran V, Schentag C, Gladman DD. **Are the CASPAR criteria for psoriatic arthritis accurate when applied to patients attending a family practice clinic?** *Arthritis and Rheumatism* **54**[Abstracts Supplement], F93. 2006.

34. Helliwell PS. **Classification and categorisation of psoriatic arthritis.** *Future Rheumatology* 2006; **1**(4):501–509.

4
Imaging

Ai Lyn Tan and Dennis McGonagle

Psoriatic arthritis (PsA) is classified as one of the spondyloarthropathies (SpAs), sharing similar characteristics such as involvement of the spine, sacroiliac joints, and enthesis. In addition, PsA commonly leads to a number of characteristic abnormalities either adjacent to or within synovial joints including periostitis, new bone formation, osteolysis, and distinctive changes such as the 'pencil-in-cup' deformity. The spectrum of arthritis associated with PsA can lead to disability that is equally severe to that seen in rheumatoid arthritis (RA). From a historic perspective these features were best seen on conventional radiography, especially in well-established PsA, but are often absent in early disease. Nevertheless, these characteristics are useful in differentiating PsA from other forms of inflammatory arthritis, such as RA, as these conditions may often present similarly in the clinical setting.

Like other inflammatory arthropathies, there is increasing interest in the development of more targeted and effective therapy for PsA. With potent biologic therapies (particularly anti-tumor necrosis factor [TNF] therapy) being used more frequently [1], there is a need for more sensitive and reliable methods of evaluating PsA, not only as a means of diagnosis, but also in following up patients on therapy [2]. Although conventional radiography is still the investigation of choice in the diagnosis and classification of PsA [3–5], magnetic resonance imaging (MRI) is assuming an increasingly important role in the evaluation of this disease. For example, sacroiliitis can be recognized by conventional radiography, computed tomography (CT), and MRI; however, radiography is generally relatively insensitive in detecting changes, and CT is unable to detect early onset of

sacroiliitis, which will limit its diagnostic utility in early disease [6]. Ultrasonography is unable to assess the sacroiliac joints adequately due to the inaccessibility of the joint. Only one study has shown the use of color and duplex Doppler sonography in identifying active sacroiliitis and its use in monitoring therapy [7]. On the other hand, MRI can identify early stages of sacroiliitis [8] and may aid in the early diagnosis of PsA, but validation studies are ongoing. Another hallmark of the SpA, and therefore PsA, is enthesitis, which is inflammation of the attachment of ligaments, capsule, or tendons to bones. Enthesitis is a feature that is useful in the diagnosis of PsA, and can be detected at an early stage on MRI and ultrasonography, but not on conventional radiography.

MRI also has an important role in increasing our understanding of the mechanisms of synovitis and bone damage in PsA. MRI has demonstrated a close relationship between enthesitis and adjacent osteitis, and the abnormality is greater in patients who are positive for human leukocyte antigen (HLA)-B27 [9]. Distal interphalangeal joint arthropathy is unique to PsA; MRI has demonstrated its pathology as entheseal and capsular based [9].

The drawback of MRI is its cost and availability. While conventional radiography is relatively inexpensive and more readily available, it involves radiation, as does CT; MRI and ultrasonography do not involve any ionizing radiation.

This chapter highlights the role of imaging in PsA, mixing the old with the new by initially showing the characteristic radiographic features of PsA before showing some ultrasound and MRI features of the disease, with a brief mention on CT and bone scintigraphy in PsA.

Plain radiographs of patients with arthritis mutilans

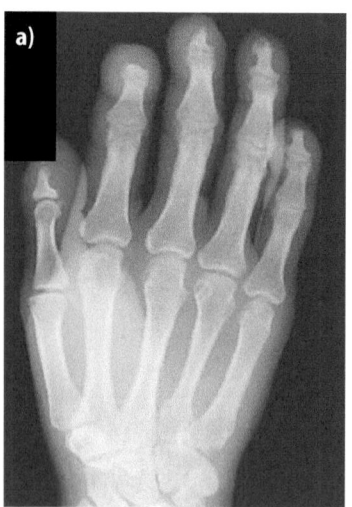

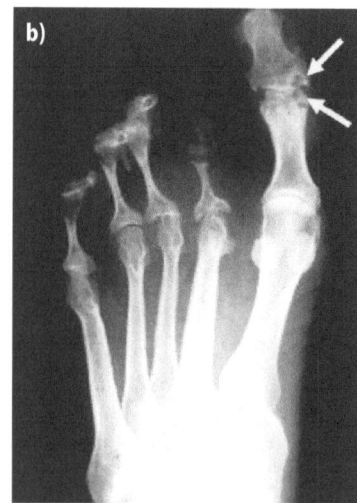

FIGURE 4.1. (a) Hand of a patient with chronic psoriatic arthritis (PsA), showing arthritis mutilans of the first to the fifth distal phalanges. The distal interphalangeal (DIP) joints are commonly affected in PsA with simultaneous involvement of the fingernail of the affected joint with dystrophy, pitting, or frank onycholysis [10,11]. This is in contrast to rheumatoid arthritis (RA) where diffuse osteoporosis, usually without osteolysis, is evident. This example shows severe osteolysis in the face of good preservation of bone mineral density elsewhere. DIP joint involvement and arthritis mutilans form two of the five subtypes of PsA as classified by Moll and Wright [12]. Arthritis mutilans of the hand is usually synonymous with DIP disease, but not all patients with DIP involvement have mutilating arthritis. The other three subtypes include polyarthritis, asymmetric oligoarthritis, and spondylitic PsA. **(b)** Another case of arthritis mutilans, in this case on a plain radiograph of the foot of a different patient, most clearly demonstrated as osteolysis of the second digit. Bone damage is also evident here, with four erosions on the first metatarsophalangeal (MTP) joint (arrows).

Plain radiograph of 'whittling' in PsA

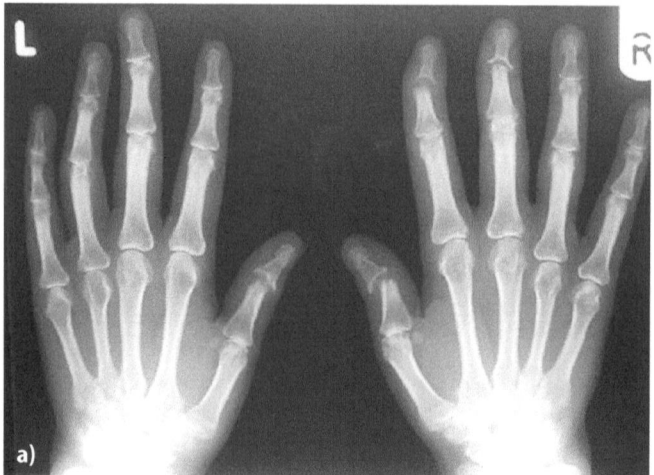

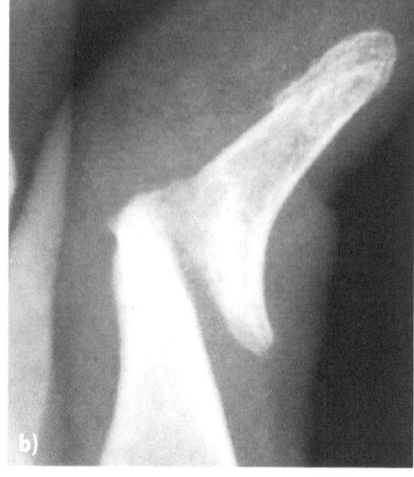

FIGURE 4.2. (a) Plain radiograph of the hands of a patient with PsA, showing classic 'pencil-in-cup' deformity in the DIP joints of the right index and middle fingers and the interphalangeal joints of the thumbs, with radial subluxation of the distal phalange of the right thumb. The deformity is a result of expansion of the base of the distal phalange or acrolysis or 'whittling' of the head of the phalange. Whittling is derived from the verb 'to whittle', which means to pare something down or taper it to a point. **(b)** Plain radiograph of a thumb showing 'whittling' of the head of the proximal phalange. In more advanced cases, an 'opera glass' digit develops, with telescoping of the skin over the resorbed joint.

FIGURE 4.3. Classic periostitis with periosteal new bone formation as a result of osteoblastic activity (arrow heads) is evident on the proximal phalange; an erosion is also seen on the head of the proximal phalange (arrow). There is osteolysis of the distal phalange. Periosteal new bone formation tends to be close to and parallel to the cortex of phalanges, metacarpals, and metatarsal [13]. When there is new bone formation as well as increased bone mineralization of the phalange, it is known as an 'ivory phalange' [14]. This patient was able to demonstrate telescoping of the DIP joint, and the overlapping skin of the DIP joint is just visible on the radiograph.

Plain radiograph of characteristic changes in finger in chronic PsA – classic periostitis

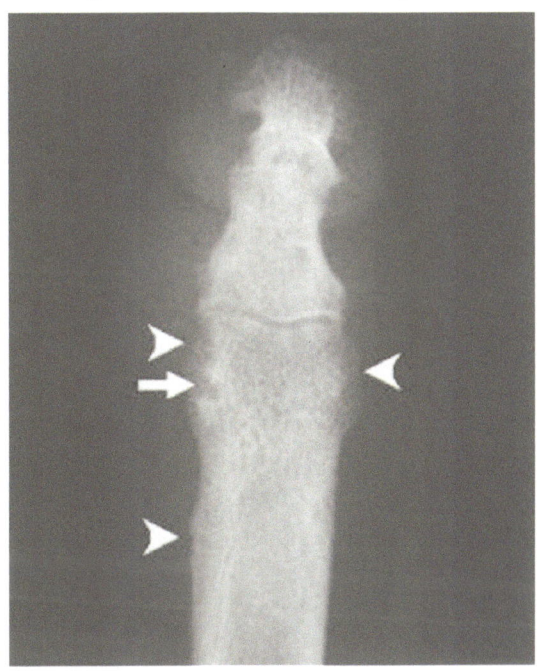

Inflammatory polyarthritis in chronic PsA

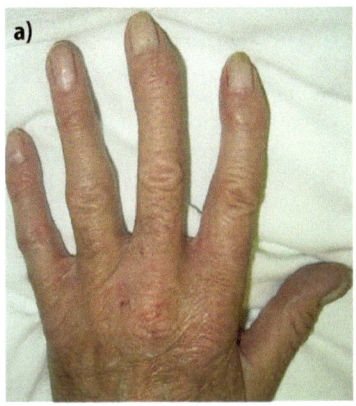

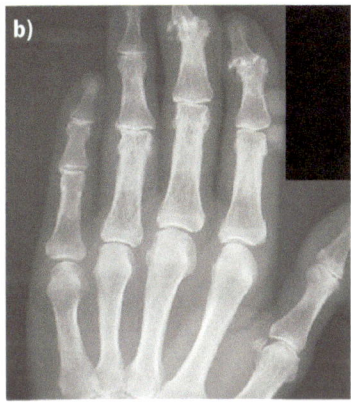

FIGURE 4.4. Many patients with psoriasis and arthritis have an inflammatory polyarthritis with small joint involvement but without joint osteolysis. **(a)** Subluxation of the second and third DIP joints is evident in this patient with chronic PsA who also had pitting of his nails. **(b)** Plain radiography shows the markedly abnormal second and third DIP joints with subluxation of both joints toward the ulnar side, loss of joint space, subchondral bone sclerosis, and formation of enthesophytes on the ulnar side representing an enthesitis related pathology at that site. DIP joint involvement affects 5–10% of patients with PsA; radiographically, PsA can resemble the changes of an osteoarthritic joint.

Multiple peri-articular bone erosions in PsA patient receiving combination therapy

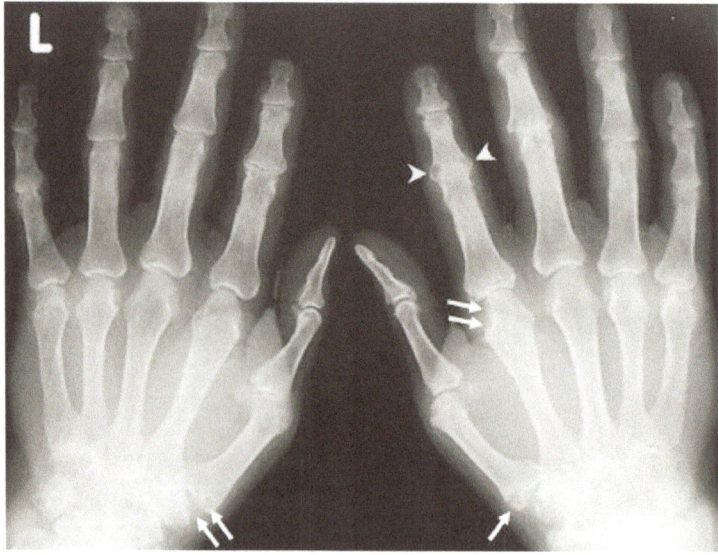

FIGURE 4.5. Plain radiograph of the hands of a patient with PsA who was being treated with a combination of methotrexate and sulphasalazine, the most commonly used disease-modifying agents in the management of PsA. Periarticular bone erosions are evident at multiple sites (arrows), including the second metacarpophalangeal (MCP) head on the right hand and the base of both thumbs. However, unlike RA and osteoarthritis where similar patterns of erosions are evident at the MCP joint or the base of the thumb, respectively, a number of other characteristic PsA-related changes are evident, including the asymmetric pattern of the MCP joint erosion and entheseal new bone formation about the second proximal interphalangeal (PIP) joint of the right hand (arrow heads). There is also loss of joint space and periostitis of the third PIP joint on the right hand.

PsA with rheumatoid-like features – ulnar deviation of the MCP joints

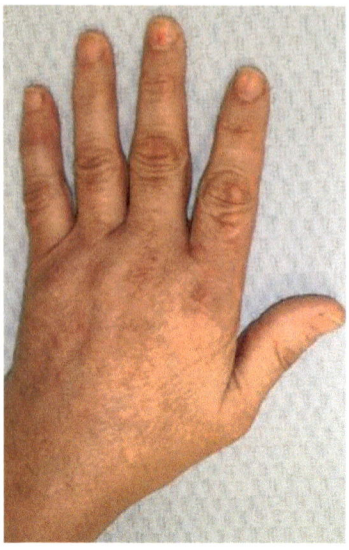

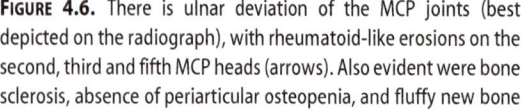

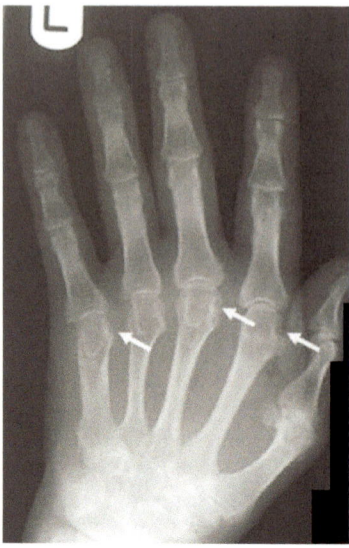

FIGURE 4.6. There is ulnar deviation of the MCP joints (best depicted on the radiograph), with rheumatoid-like erosions on the second, third and fifth MCP heads (arrows). Also evident were bone sclerosis, absence of periarticular osteopenia, and fluffy new bone formation about the eroded carpal bones in the wrist. There are similar changes in the distal radioulnar joint with additional new bone formation at that site.

PsA with rheumatoid-like features – fibular deviation of the toes

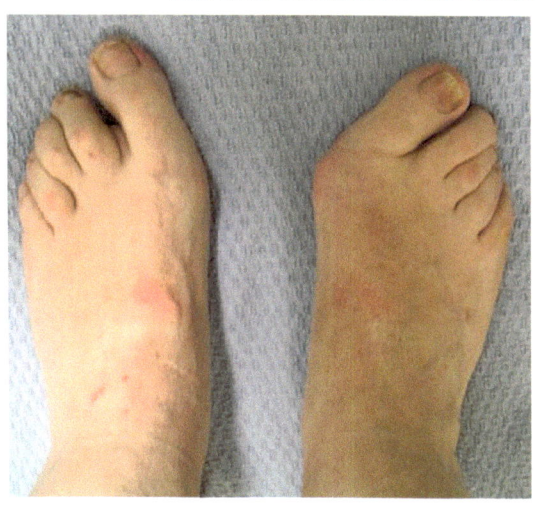 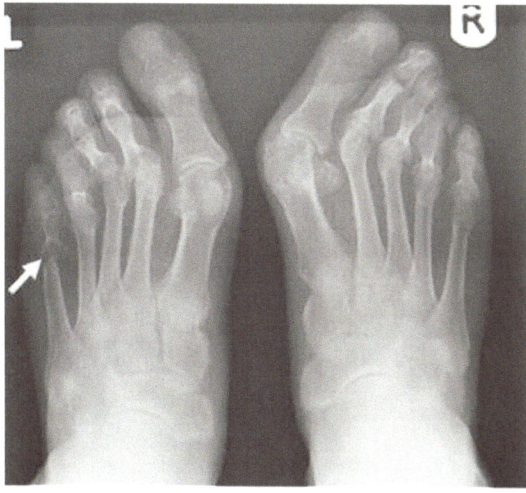

FIGURE 4.7. Feet of the same patient shown in Figure 4.6 demonstrating fibular deviation of the toes. Although the pattern of polyarticular disease is reminiscent of RA, the radiograph is characteristic of PsA with joint fusion or ankylosis at several sites, lack of osteopenia and a characteristic 'pencil-in-cup'-type deformity at the fifth MTP joint on the left (arrow), with proximal joint osteolysis and distal joint new bone formation at the capsule. The entheseal bone formation at the distal capsule forms the cup in the 'pencil-in-cup' deformity of the fifth MTP joint on the left foot. This case illustrates how a disease pattern that appears to be primarily synovial-based on clinical findings can in fact be associated with enthesitis and bone-based pathology on radiographic findings. Some patients classified as PsA polyarthritis have juxta-articular osteoporosis and erosions only and no evidence of an enthesitis/osteitis-related pathology. Concerns about diagnosing such patients with PsA have been raised.

Monoarthritis of the right wrist in patient with PsA

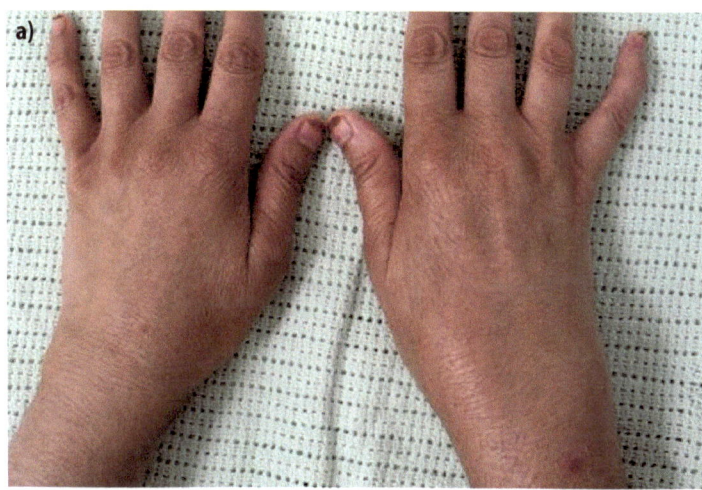 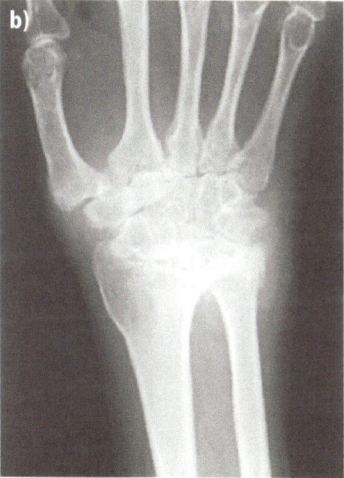

FIGURE 4.8. **(a)** The right wrist of this 38-year-old female is clinically swollen. **(b)** Plain radiograph of the right wrist of the patient. There is loss of joint space among the carpal bones as well as between the radius and ulna and the carpal bones. Bone mineralization is relatively well preserved unlike in RA, where there is often periarticular osteoporosis. Involvement of the wrist and hand is seen in 75% of patients with PsA [15]; although the wrist is less frequently affected than the hands, it can often present as a monoarthritis or as part of an oligoarthritis in PsA. Monoarthritis or oligoarthritis are the most common presenting patterns in PsA [16], and form one of the patterns of involvement in PsA described by Moll and Wright, where asymmetric distribution of joint involvement is characteristic [12,17].

Syndesmophytes in PsA

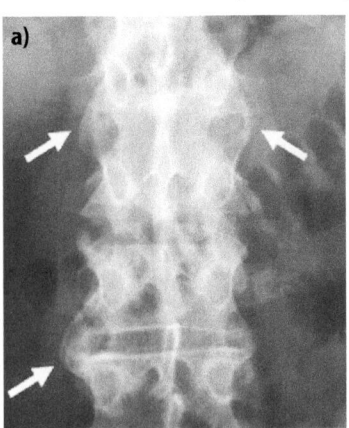

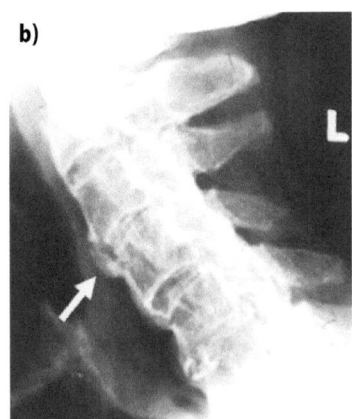

FIGURE 4.9. One of the main pathologies affecting the spine in PsA is the development of syndesmophytes. These paravertebral ossifications tend to be non- marginal or chunky syndesmophytes. Unlike the marginal syndesmophytes found in ankylosing spondylitis, the chunky syndesmophytes in PsA tend to be sparse and asymmetrically distributed. (a) Coronal view of plain radiograph of the lumbar spine of a patient with chronic PsA showing chunky syndesmophytes (arrows). (b) Plain radiograph showing lateral view of the cervical spine of a different patient with PsA with syndesmophytes (arrow). The cervical spine is frequently involved in PsA [18]. The most common radiographic changes in the cervical spine are apophyseal joint ankylosis and anterior atlantoaxial joint subluxation [19].

Enthesophytes in PsA

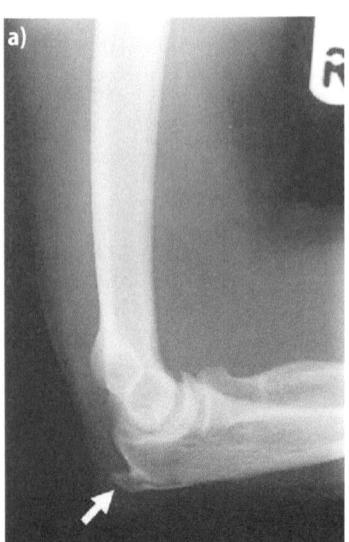

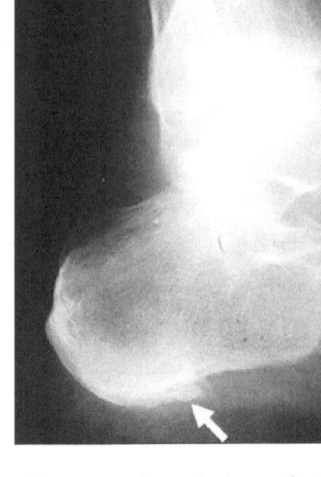

FIGURE 4.10. (a) Plain radiograph of the right elbow of a patient with PsA showing an enthesophyte at the triceps insertion. (b) Plain radiograph of the calcaneum of a different patient with PsA showing an enthesophyte (arrow) where the plantar fascia attaches, more commonly known as a calcaneal spur. An enthesis is where tendons, ligaments, or joint capsules attach to bones. The inflammation of an enthesis or enthesitis is an important concept in PsA, commonly leading toward the formation of new bone at the enthesis, or enthesophytes [9]. Understanding the pathogenesis of enthesitis has important implications in the diagnosis and treatment of PsA [20].

Ultrasonographs showing capsular edema in PsA

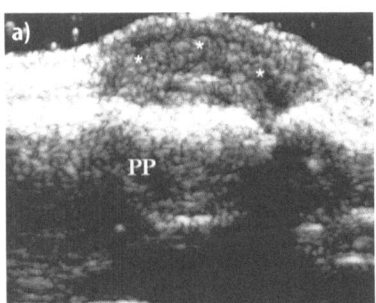 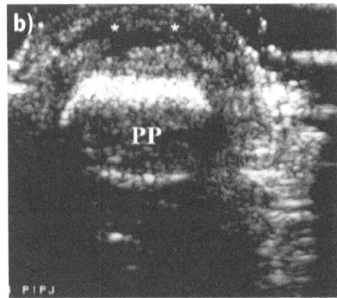 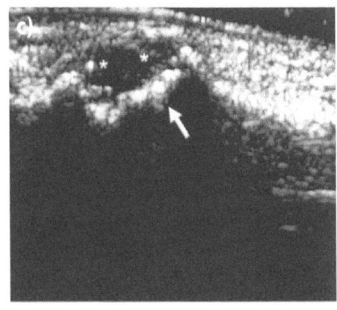

FIGURE 4.11. **(a)** Longitudinal view of the third PIP joint of a patient with early PsA showing capsular edema or synovitis (asterisks). **(b)** Transverse view of the same joint showing capsular edema (asterisks). **(c)** Ultrasonograph of a different patient who was diagnosed with PsA 6 months earlier. There is entheseal calcification at the fourth PIP joint (arrow). There was also edema within the capsule (asterisks).

Ultrasonography is suited to the study of small joints, such as the finger joints, as the structures within are relatively superficial. The advantage of ultrasonography over plain radiography is that it does not involve ionizing radiation and is capable of real-time scanning. It is relatively inexpensive and easily available, and is suited for the study of small peripheral joints and superficial structures. PP, proximal phalange.

Ultrasonography of patellar tendon enthesitis in PsA

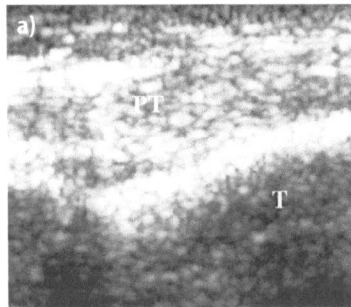 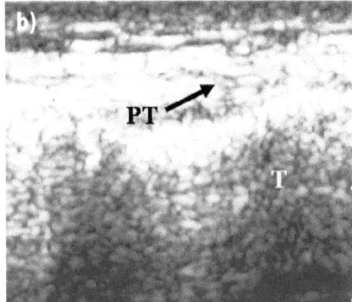

FIGURE 4.12. **(a)** Ultrasonograph of the right knee of a patient with PsA showing hypoechoic thickening of the insertion and loss of definition of the edge of the patellar tendon (PT). **(b)** The contralateral uninvolved PT insertion is shown for comparison. As already mentioned, enthesitis is a hallmark of PsA, and forms part of the diagnostic criteria for SpA [21]. Enthesitis may be difficult to detect clinically, and ultrasonography has been shown to be better at detecting enthesitis in the lower limbs of patients with SpA [22]. The use of ultrasonography, including power Doppler, has been shown to be useful in both the diagnosis and assessment of activity in SpA [23].

Ultrasonographs of plantar fasciitis and patellar tendonitis

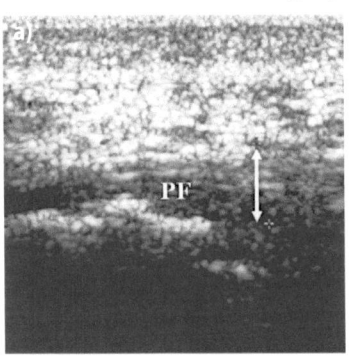 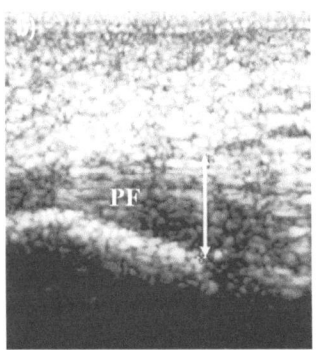 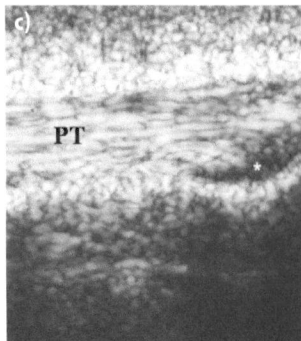

FIGURE 4.13. This patient with PsA was symptomatic in both feet and the left knee. **(a,b)** Right plantar fascia (PF) (left panel) and left PF of the patient demonstrating plantar fasciitis (center panel). There was loss of the fibrillar pattern of the PF bilaterally, and a markedly thickened PF on the left (double-headed arrows). **(c)** Sagittal view of the left PT with a bursa near the insertion or enthesis (asterisk). Although inflammation can occur at any enthesis in PsA, enthesitis tends to be more common in the lower limbs [24]. Ultrasonography is able to provide more information than clinical examination of enthesitis [25], and, therefore, can help with the diagnosis of PsA. There is a need for validation of ultrasonography in the diagnosis of PsA.

Ultrasonography and MRI of plantar faciitis in PsA

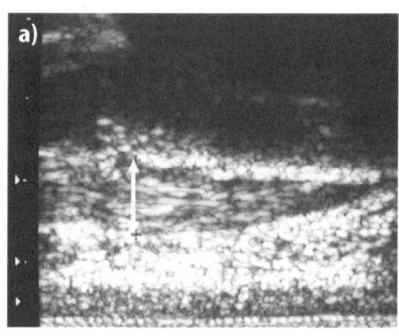 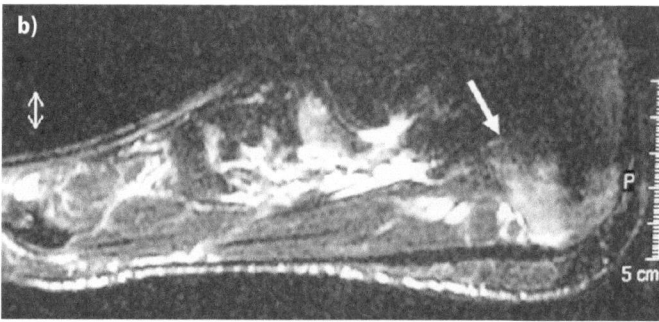

FIGURE 4.14. (a) Ultrasonograph from a 37-year-old female with PsA showing hypoechoic thickening of the PF (double-headed arrow), measuring 0.44 cm thick (each mark on the scale on the left represents 0.5 cm). (b) T2-weighted fat-suppressed magnetic resonance imaging (MRI) showing associated adjacent bone edema on the calcaneum depicted by high signal (arrow). Plantar fasciitis is an enthesitis, and is common in PsA. Rarely, it can be the presenting feature of PsA [26]. Effective therapy of enthesitis by biologic blockade has been successfully demonstrated on power Doppler sonography, which measures the vascularity or inflammation within the enthesis [27].

MRI of the hands in PsA – capsular-based edema

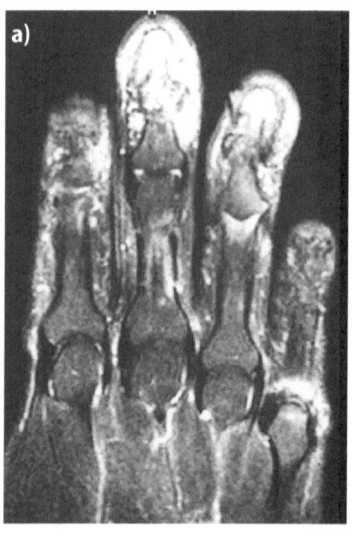 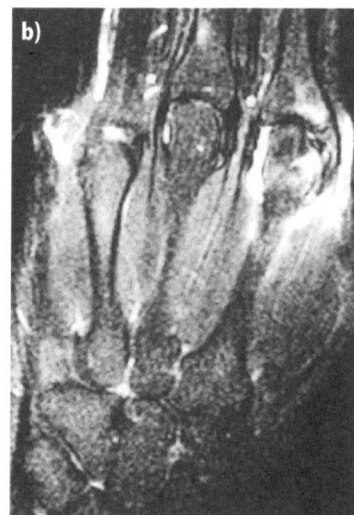

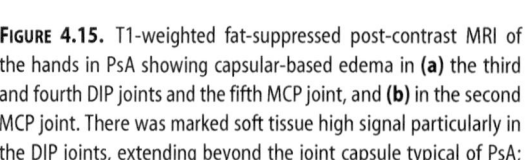

FIGURE 4.15. T1-weighted fat-suppressed post-contrast MRI of the hands in PsA showing capsular-based edema in (a) the third and fourth DIP joints and the fifth MCP joint, and (b) in the second MCP joint. There was marked soft tissue high signal particularly in the DIP joints, extending beyond the joint capsule typical of PsA; high signal was also detected in the second MCP joint (b). MRI has been used to monitor response to therapy in PsA, and has determined the effectiveness of biologic agents in reducing inflammation in this disease [28].

Use of MRI in early PsA

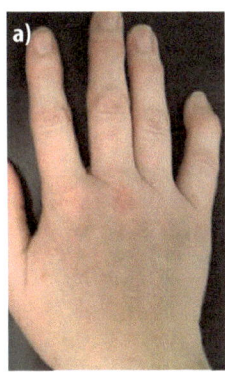 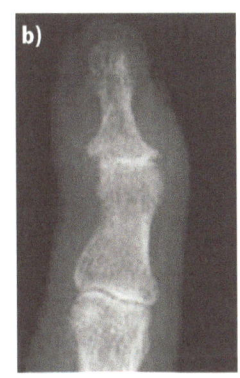 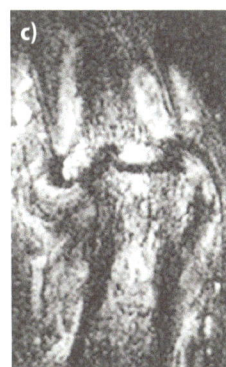

FIGURE 4.16. **(a)** A patient with PsA who had an 8-month history of symptomatic DIP joint involvement in the little finger showing ankylosis of the joint. **(b)** Plain radiograph of the same joint showing subluxation and loss of joint space. **(c)** On T2-weighted fat-suppressed high-resolution MRI we can see bone edema depicted by a high signal, particularly near the joint and the enthesis where the collateral ligaments insert. The advantages of MRI over plain radiography in PsA include absence of ionizing radiation, the ability to perform multiplanar imaging, the ability to detect inflammation, and better sensitivity in early disease [6]. In addition, high-resolution MRI using specialised MRI 'microscopy coils', ideal for examination of small joints like in the fingers, has allowed us to identify micro-anatomical differences between PsA and osteoarthritis of the DIP joint [29].

MRI of knee of HLA-B27-positive patient with PsA

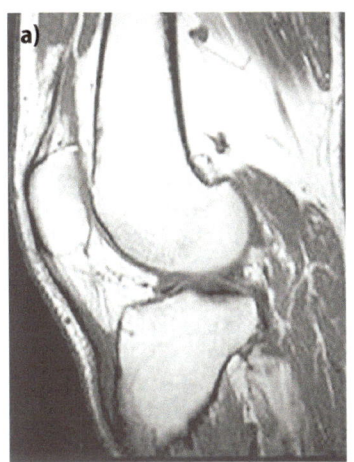 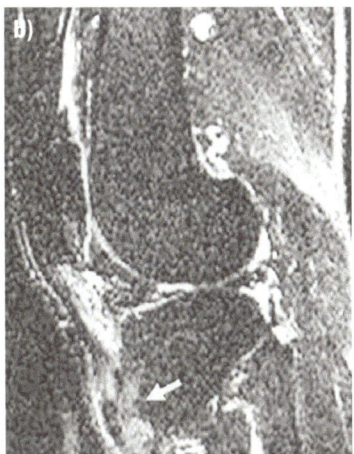 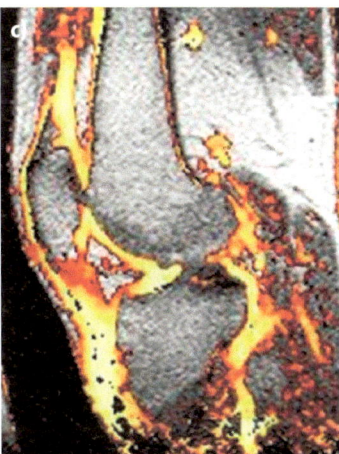

FIGURE 4.17. **(a)** T1-weighted sagittal image of the knee delineating the anatomy of the joint. **(b)** T2-weighted fat-suppressed sagittal image of the knee showing sites of inflammation indicated by high signal. **(c)** Dynamic post-contrast MRI with gadolinium diethylenetriamine pentaacetic acid. The image was postprocessed with commercial software (Analyze®; Mayo Clinics, New York, USA) and software developed in-house [30]. The colors on the image signify areas of relative vascularity or inflammation, with yellow representing areas of greater inflammation and red indicating milder inflammation. Using this method of analysis, it has been found that the area of synovitis in SpA, of which PsA is a part, is greater than that found in RA [31]. However, like RA, there is a significant variation in synovitis within the knee, with greater synovitis demonstrated at the cartilage pannus junction compared to that at the more proximal suprapatellar pouch [31]. This image also shows enthesitis at the PT insertion depicted as edema adjacent to the attachment site and also within the bone (arrow). Enthesitis within or adjacent to synovial joints is a prominent feature of early PsA-related synovial joint disease and it may be clinically unrecognizable.

MRI of patient with SAPHO syndrome

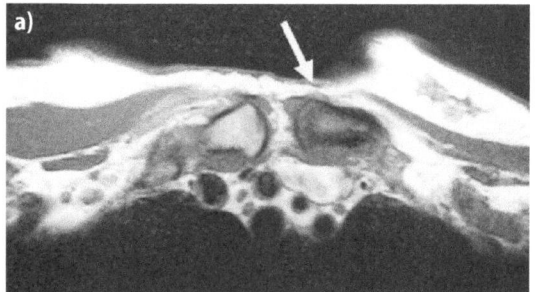

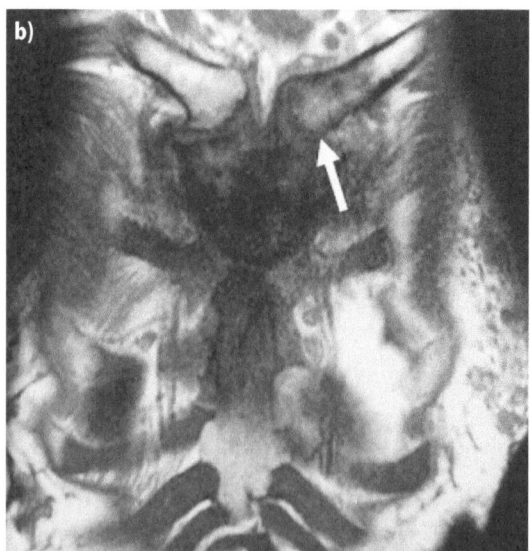

FIGURE 4.18. A characteristic arthropathy associated with PsA is the SAPHO syndrome, which stands for synovitis, acne, pustulosis, hyperostosis, and osteitis. This arthropathy most typically involves the sternoclavicular joint (65–90% of SAPHO patients), but one or more sites can be affected [32]. While there has been much debate about the classification of SAPHO in relation to PsA, MRI shows a similar mechanism (especially prominent osteitis) to disease at other sites. **(a)** Axial and **(b)** coronal T1-weighted MRIs of the sternoclavicular joint in a patient with SAPHO syndrome who had pain and tenderness over the left sternoclavicular joint. On T1-weighted images the osteitis has a low signal (arrows). Following a course of intravenous pamidronate, the patient improved symptomatically.

Scintigraphy and MRI of patient with SAPHO syndrome

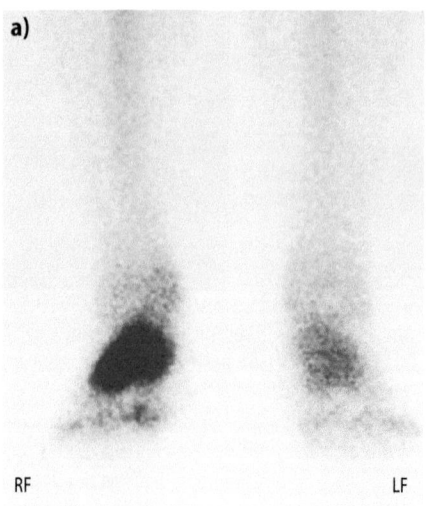

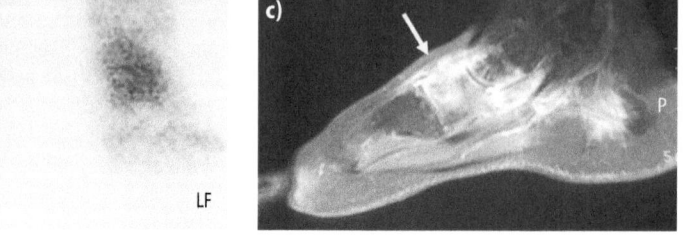

FIGURE 4.19. A characteristic feature of PsA on scintigraphy is prominent tracer uptake within the bones [33]. Bone scintigraphy was once thought to be the most important imaging tool in PsA; although it is more sensitive than plain radiography, its limitation renders it too unspecific to aid diagnosis. **(a)** This bone scan shows high tracer uptake in the right midfoot of a patient with SAPHO syndrome, which is associated with PsA. Peripheral joint involve-ment has been reported in up to 36% of SAPHO patients [34]. The MRIs show anatomic sites of inflammation with tendonitis, synovitis, and cuboid and medial cuneiform bone edema. These appear dark (arrow) on the T1-weighted MRI **(b)** and appear as highlights (arrow) on the post-contrast MRI **(c)**. This pattern of diffuse inflammation is characteristic of SpA and PsA and is seen at other sites, including the sacroiliac joints. LF, left foot; RF, right foot.

Imaging of sacroiliac joints of patient with HLA-B27-positive PsA

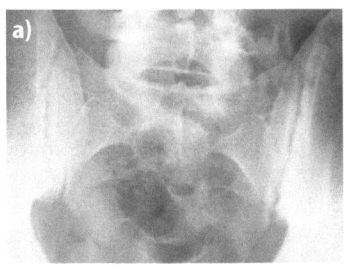 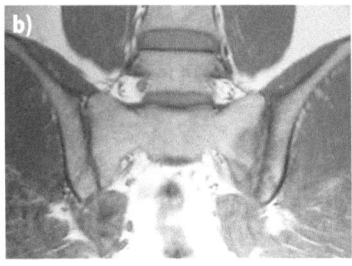 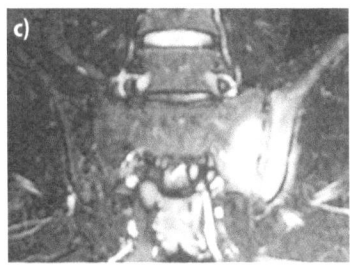

FIGURE 4.20. (a) The plain radiograph shows an almost normal appearance of the sacroiliac joints. **(b)** T1-weighted MRI scan showing sacroiliitis on the left side, appearing dark. **(c)** T2-weighted fat-suppressed post-contrast MRI scan showing high signal over the left sacroiliac joint on both the sacral and iliac sides indicating marked bone marrow edema that is thought to be related to an osteitis. Sacroiliitis occurs in 10–25% of patients with PsA [35], but radiographic sacroiliitis has been reported in up to 78% of patients with PsA [36]. Asymmetric sacroiliitis is more common in PsA than in ankylosing spondylitis, as in this case [18]. HLA-B27 positivity has been found to be associated with earlier onset and greater severity of sacroiliitis, as well as development of bilateral sacroiliitis [37–39]. The radiographic changes of sacroiliitis are often not detectable in early disease; however, MRI is able to show early signs of sacroiliitis indicated by bone marrow edema at the joint.

CT scan of pelvis of PsA patient showing sacroiliitis

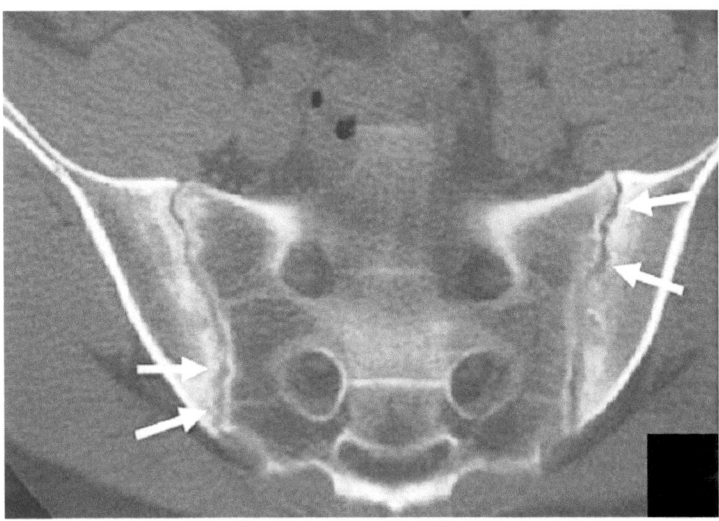

FIGURE 4.21. CT scan showing sacroiliitis, with erosions (arrows) and sclerosis, mainly on the iliac part of the joint and irregular joint space. CT is superior to plain radiography and bone scintigraphy in evaluating sacroiliitis, but should be used only as an adjunct to radiography in equivocal cases to confirm sacroiliitis [35]. Both CT and MRI are capable of detecting sacroiliitis in early disease, before radiographic changes are evident; however, MRI is able to identify inflammatory changes of the sacroiliac joint before any changes are visible on CT and, unlike CT, MRI does not involve any ionizing radiation [40]. In addition, the degree of enhancement on dynamic MRI has been found to be correlated with the cellularity of T-cells and macrophages in early and active SpA, confirming MRI as a reliable imaging modality in early disease [41].

References

1. Barry J, Kirby B. **Novel biologic therapies for psoriasis.** *Expert Opin Biol Ther* 2004; **4**:975–987.
2. McGonagle D. **Diagnosis and treatment of enthesitis.** *Rheum Dis Clin North Am* 2003; **29**:549–560.
3. Taylor WJ, Porter GG, Helliwell PS. **Operational definitions and observer reliability of the plain radiographic features of psoriatic arthritis.** *J Rheumatol* 2003; **30**:2645–2658.
4. McGonagle D, Conaghan PG, Emery P. **Psoriatic arthritis: a unified concept twenty years on.** *Arthritis Rheum* 1999; **42**:1080–1086.
5. Fournie B, Crognier L, Arnaud C *et al.* **Proposed classification criteria of psoriatic arthritis. A preliminary study in 260 patients.** *Rev Rheum* 1999; **66**:446–456.
6. Tan AL, Wakefield RJ, Conaghan PG *et al.* **Imaging of the musculoskeletal system: magnetic resonance imaging, ultrasonography and computed tomography.** *Best Pract Res Clin Rheumatol* 2003; **17**:513–528.
7. Arslan H, Sakarya ME, Adak B *et al.* **Duplex and color Doppler sonographic findings in active sacroiliitis.** *Am J Roentgenol* 1999; **173**:677–680.
8. Williamson L, Dockerty JL, Dalbeth N *et al.* **Clinical assessment of sacroiliitis and HLA-B27 are poor predictors of sacroiliitis diagnosed by magnetic resonance imaging in psoriatic arthritis.** *Rheumatology* 2004; **43**:85–88.
9. McGonagle D, Marzo-Ortega H, Benjamin M *et al.* **Report on the Second International Enthesitis Workshop.** *Arthritis Rheum* 2003; **48**:896–905.
10. Scarpa R, Manguso F, Oriente A *et al.* **Is the involvement of the distal interphalangeal joint in psoriatic patients related to nail psoriasis?** *Clin Rheumatol* 2004; **23**:27–30.
11. Williamson L, Dalbeth N, Dockerty JL *et al.* **Extended report: nail disease in psoriatic arthritis – clinically important, potentially treatable and often overlooked.** *Rheumatology* 2004; **43**:790–794.
12. Moll JM, Wright V. **Psoriatic arthritis.** *Semin Arthritis Rheum* 1973; **3**:55–78.
13. Forrester DM, Kirkpatrick J. **Periostitis and pseudoperiostitis.** *Radiology* 1976; **118**:597–601.
14. Resnick D, Broderick TW. **Bony proliferation of terminal toe phalanges in psoriasis: the 'ivory' phalanx.** *J Can Assoc Radiol* 1977; **28**:187–189.
15. Martel W, Stuck KJ, Dworin AM *et al.* **Erosive osteoarthritis and psoriatic arthritis: a radiologic comparison in the hand, wrist, and foot.** *Am J Roentgenol* 1980; **134**:125–135.
16. Marsal S, Armadans-Gil L, Martinez M *et al.* **Clinical, radiographic and HLA associations as markers for different patterns of psoriatic arthritis.** *Rheumatology* 1999; **38**:332–337.
17. Jones SM, Armas JB, Cohen MG *et al.* **Psoriatic arthritis: outcome of disease subsets and relationship of joint disease to nail and skin disease.** *Br J Rheumatol* 1994; **33**:834–839.
18. Helliwell PS, Hickling P, Wright V. **Do the radiological changes of classic ankylosing spondylitis differ from the changes found in the spondylitis associated with inflammatory bowel disease, psoriasis, and reactive arthritis?** *Ann Rheum Dis* 1998; **57**:135–140.
19. Laiho K, Kauppi M. **The cervical spine in patients with psoriatic arthritis.** *Ann Rheum Dis* 2002; **61**:650–652.
20. McGonagle D, Benjamin M, Marzo-Ortega H *et al.* **Advances in the understanding of entheseal inflammation.** *Curr Rheumatol Rep* 2002; **4**:500–506.
21. Dougados M, van der Linden S, Juhlin R *et al.* **The European Spondylarthropathy Study Group preliminary criteria for the classification of spondylarthropathy.** *Arthritis Rheum* 1991; **34**:1218–1227.
22. Balint PV, Kane D, Wilson H *et al.* **Ultrasonography of entheseal insertions in the lower limb in spondyloarthropathy.** *Ann Rheum Dis* 2002; **61**:905–910.
23. D'Agostino MA, Said-Nahal R, Hacquard-Bouder C *et al.* **Assessment of peripheral enthesitis in the spondylarthropathies by ultrasonography combined with power Doppler: a cross-sectional study.** *Arthritis Rheum* 2003; **48**:523–533.
24. McGonagle D, Khan MA, Marzo-Ortega H *et al.* **Enthesitis in spondyloarthropathy.** *Curr Opin Rheumatol* 1999; **11**:244–250.
25. Lehtinen A, Taavitsainen M, Leirisalo-Repo M. **Sonographic analysis of enthesopathy in the lower extremities of patients with spondylarthropathy.** *Clin Exp Rheumatol* 1994; **12**:143–148.
26. Scarpa R. **Peripheral enthesopathies in psoriatic arthritis.** *J Rheumatol* 1998; **25**:2288–2289.
27. D'Agostino MA, Breban M, Said-Nahal R *et al.* **Refractory inflammatory heel pain in spondylarthropathy: a significant response to infliximab documented by ultrasound.** *Arthritis Rheum* 2002; **46**:840–841. Author reply 841–843.
28. Antoni C, Dechant C, Hanns-Martin Lorenz PD *et al.* **Open-label study of infliximab treatment for psoriatic arthritis: clinical and magnetic resonance imaging measurements of reduction of inflammation.** *Arthritis Rheum* 2002; **47**:506–512.
29. Tan AL, Grainger AJ, Tanner SF *et al.* **A high-resolution magnetic resonance imaging study of distal interphalangeal joint arthropathy in psori-

atic arthritis and osteoarthritis: are they the same? *Arthritis Rheum* 2006; **54**:1328–1333.

30. Reece RJ, Kraan MC, Radjenovic A *et al.* Comparative assessment of leflunomide and methotrexate for the treatment of rheumatoid arthritis, by dynamic enhanced magnetic resonance imaging. *Arthritis Rheum* 2002; **46**:366–372.

31. Rhodes LA, Tan AL, Tanner SF *et al.* Regional variation and differential response to therapy of knee synovitis adjacent to the cartilage pannus junction and suprapatellar pouch in inflammatory arthritis: Implications for pathogenesis and therapy of inflammatory arthritis. *Arthritis Rheum* 2004; **50**:2428–2432.

32. Earwaker JW, Cotten A. SAPHO: syndrome or concept? Imaging findings. *Skeletal Radiol* 2003; **32**:311–327.

33. Marchesoni A, Helliwell P, Gallazzi M *et al.* Psoriatic arthritis in British and Italian patients: a comparative clinical, radiologic, and scintigraphic study. *J Rheumatol* 1999; **26**:2619–2621.

34. Hayem G, Bouchaud-Chabot A, Benali K *et al.* SAPHO syndrome: a long-term follow-up study of 120 cases. *Semin Arthritis Rheum* 1999; **29**:159–171.

35. Salonen DC, Brower AC *et al.* Seronegative spondyloarthropathies: imaging. In: *Rheumatology.* Edited by MC Hochberg, AJ Silman, JS Smolen. Philadelphia: Mosby, 2003; 1193–1204.

36. Battistone MJ, Manaster BJ, Reda DJ *et al.* The prevalence of sacroilitis in psoriatic arthritis: new perspectives from a large, multicenter cohort. A Department of Veterans Affairs Cooperative Study. *Skeletal Radiol* 1999; **28**:196–201.

37. Puhakka KB, Jurik AG, Schiottz-Christensen B *et al.* Magnetic resonance imaging of sacroiliitis in early seronegative spondylarthropathy. Abnormalities correlated to clinical and laboratory findings. *Rheumatology* 2004; **43**:234–237.

38. Queiro R, Sarasqueta C, Belzunegui J *et al.* Psoriatic spondyloarthropathy: a comparative study between HLA-B27 positive and HLA-B27 negative disease. *Semin Arthritis Rheum* 2002; **31**:413–418.

39. Tsai YG, Chang DM, Kuo SY *et al.* Relationship between human lymphocyte antigen-B27 and clinical features of psoriatic arthritis. *J Microbiol Immunol Infect* 2003; **36**:101–104.

40. Braun J, Sieper J. The sacroiliac joint in the spondyloarthropathies. *Curr Opin Rheumatol* 1996; **8**:275–287.

41. Bollow M, Fischer T, Reisshauer H *et al.* Quantitative analyses of sacroiliac biopsies in spondyloarthropathies: T cells and macrophages predominate in early and active sacroiliitis – cellularity correlates with the degree of enhancement detected by magnetic resonance imaging. *Ann Rheum Dis* 2000; **59**:135–140.

5
Skin and Psoriasis

Kristina P. Callis and Gerald G. Krueger

Psoriasis is a chronic, inflammatory skin disease typically manifesting as well-demarcated plaques with varying degrees of erythema, scale, thickness, and body surface area affected. It is considered a heritable, T-cell-mediated autoimmune disorder. Like many genetic disorders, there is a large range of phenotypic expression, and many environmental factors, such as infection, trauma, drugs, and stress, are believed to influence the onset, course, and severity of psoriasis. Psoriasis can be extremely detrimental to the individual with significant psychosocial and medical implications. The disease is considered moderate to severe in about 30% of patients, and the most effective treatments are immunosuppressive agents and light therapy with risk of end-organ toxicity [1].

The prevalence of psoriasis is estimated to range between 1% and 3% of the general population. It occurs more commonly in the Caucasian population compared with Blacks or Asians in whom it affects less than 1%. The average age of onset is in the late 20s [2]. The age of onset of psoriasis is bimodal, the first peak prior to age 40 (type I) and the second peak after age 40 (type II) [3]. Early onset is associated with positive family history, more severe disease, and human leukocyte antigen (HLA)-Cw6 positivity [4].

Pathophysiology

Psoriasis is currently considered a T-cell-mediated autoimmune disease with a complex immunologic basis. The disease is characterized histologically by hyperproliferation of the epidermis, abnormal dif-

ferentiation of keratinocytes, and inflammation (*see* Figure 5.2). The disease is most likely initiated by an endogenous or exogenous antigen that is presented by dendritic cells to lymphocytes in regional lymph nodes [5]. Activated CD4+ and CD8+ T-lymphocytes bearing cutaneous lymphocyte antigen (CLA) allows them to bind to endothelial receptors, extravasate, and infiltrate the dermis and epidermis [6]. Further interaction with antigen-presenting dendritic cells results in inflammation mediated by cytokine release, chemokines, adhesion molecules, and growth factors. A Th1 cytokine profile, including interleukin (IL)-2, interferon-γ, and tumor necrosis factor (TNF)-α, predominates [7]. Identification of key cytokines and receptor interactions in the pathogenesis of psoriasis, such as the intercellular adhesion molecule (ICAM)-1/leukocyte function-associated antigen (LFA)-1 interaction, LFA-3/CD2 costimulatory response, production of TNF, IL-12 and IL-23, has led to the development of specific pharmacologic targets in the treatment of psoriasis [8,9].

The Psoriasis Phenotype

Psoriasis is defined as '*A chronic skin disease that is classically characterized by thickened, red areas of skin covered with silvery scales*' [10]. The diagnosis of psoriasis is nearly always clinical, taking into account the morphology of the lesions, the distribution, and associated findings such as nail disease, joint disease, precipitating events such as antecedent infections or new medications, and family history of psoriasis. Biopsies are sometimes used to exclude conditions in the differential diagnosis, including other papulosquamous disorders such as parapsoriasis, cutaneous T-cell lymphoma, and eczema.

The morphology, distribution, and extent of body surface area involvement are quite varied from individual to individual, but certain patterns of disease do predominate. Plaque or discoid-type psoriasis is the most common and easily recognized variant, occurring in more than 80% of cases. Plaques can range from thin, faintly red plaques with minimal fine scale to very thick, beefy red plaques that are covered with a thick, silvery tenacious scale. Other morphologic variants may co-exist with plaque-type disease, or manifest as the predominating form in an individual patient, including flexural or inverse, guttate, palmoplantar (pustular and non-pustular variants), generalized pustular, and erythrodermic. Guttate psoriasis occurs in about 10% of patients, with erythrodermic and pustular forms occurring in fewer than 3% [11,12].

The distribution and extent of psoriasis is also extremely varied and linked to the morphology of

disease. Classic plaque-type psoriasis will affect the scalp, ears, extensor elbows and knees, umbilicus, and sacrum. The lesions of inverse or flexural disease tend to be well-demarcated erythematous patches with little scale and a tendency to macerate and become secondarily infected. Guttate plaques are small, usually bright red but less indurated, and are widely scattered over the trunk and extremities. Erythrodermic psoriasis is manifested as widespread, red, scaling lesions with associated palmar/plantar involvement, that may be associated with fever, chills, hypotension, insensible fluid losses, and hypoalbuminemia.

The majority of patients will have scalp involvement. Typically, lesions will occur in the post-auricular scalp or at the hairline. At times the face will become involved, and may overlap with the clinical features of seborrheic dermatitis, often designated sebopsoriasis.

Nail changes are also seen in the majority of patients, ranging from minor pitting to severely disfiguring and functionally disabling dystrophy. Nail findings have been associated with distal interphalangeal psoriatic arthritis [13,14].

MHC and non-MHC psoriasis loci

Locus name	Chromosome	Candidate genes/regions
PSORS1	6p21.3	HLA-C, corneodesmosin, HCR, others [23–29]
PSORS2	17q25	RUNX1 [30] RAPTOR [31]
PSORS3	4q34	[32]
PSORS4	1q21	S100 genes in epidermal differentiation complex [33]
PSORS5	3q	[26]
PSORS6	19p13	[27]
PSORS7	1p	[28]
PSORS8	16q	[23]
PSORS9	4q31	[29]

FIGURE 5.1. Psoriasis has long been recognized as having a strong genetic component, supported by high concordance rates amongst monozygotic twins, clustering in families, and patterns of recessive and dominant modes of transmission in large cohorts [15–17]. Psoriasis was first linked to the human leukocyte antigen (HLA) region in 1972, and, subsequently, class I antigens HLA-B57, HLA-B13, HLA-Cw7, and, particularly, HLA-Cw6, were identified as conferring risk [18]. Since 1994, ten genome-wide scans have been performed identifying 19 susceptibility loci on 15 different chromosomes; however, no single gene has yet been definitively implicated in causing psoriasis [19]. The predominant susceptibility locus, PSORS1, has been replicated in many studies and narrowed to a minimal consensus region near HLA-C [20–22]. Candidate genes have been identified in the major histocompatibility complex (MHC) and non-MHC loci, but no studies have yet confirmed the functional significance of these findings.

The major psoriasis susceptibility locus on chromosome 6p21, PSORS1, has been replicated in several populations and is the most extensively studied [23–29]. Candidate genes in the immediate region have included HLA-C, corneodesmosin, HCR (helic α-helix coiled-coil rod homolog gene), SEEK1, SPR1, and OTF3, as well as the more proximal TNF-α, TAP, and MICA genes. Study of PSORS2, on chromosome 17q25, has implicated polymorphisms at a runt-related transcription factor 1 (RUNX1)-binding site and regulatory associated protein of mTOR (RAPTOR) [30,31]. The major psoriasis susceptibility locus on chromosome 4q34 is PSORS3, and on 1q21 is PSORS4 [32,33].

FIGURE 5.2. Histologically, psoriasis is characterized by hyperproliferation of the epidermis with associated dilation of blood vessels in the papillary dermis and a perivascular lymphocytic infiltrate. Early lesions may have associated spongiosis or entirely normal epidermis. As lesions evolve, classic psoriasiform or 'regular' hyperplasia develops, with thinning of suprapapillary plates and mounds of parakeratosis with neutrophils seen migrating toward the parakeratotic peaks. Intracorneal collections of neutrophils (Munroe microabscesses) are seen, with collections of both neutrophils and lymphocytes in the spinous layer (spongiform pustules of Kogoj) seen less frequently.

Histopathology of psoriasis

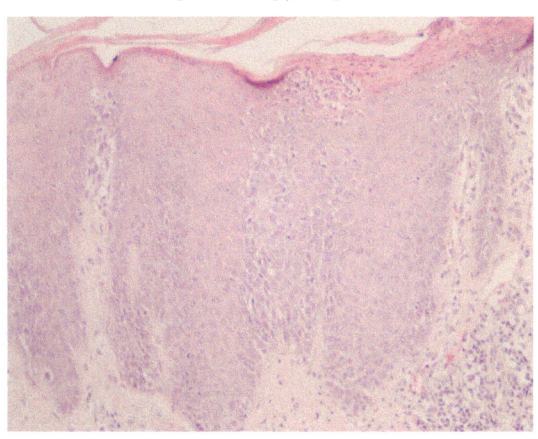

Examples of plaque-type psoriasis

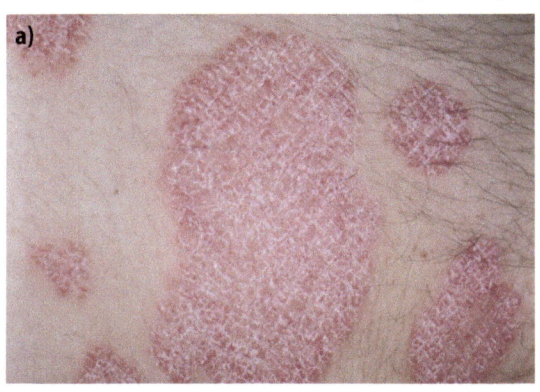

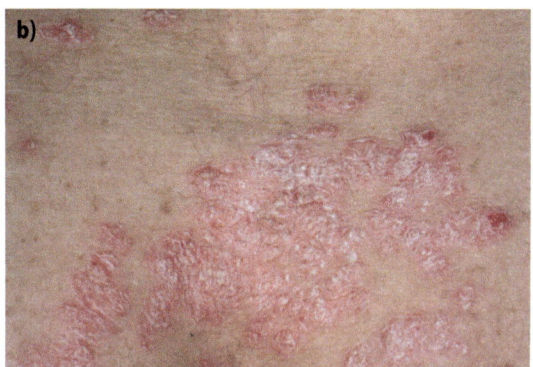

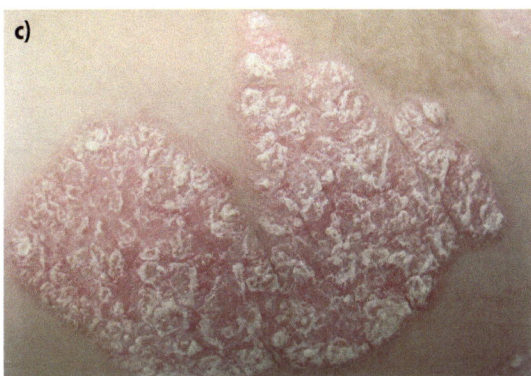

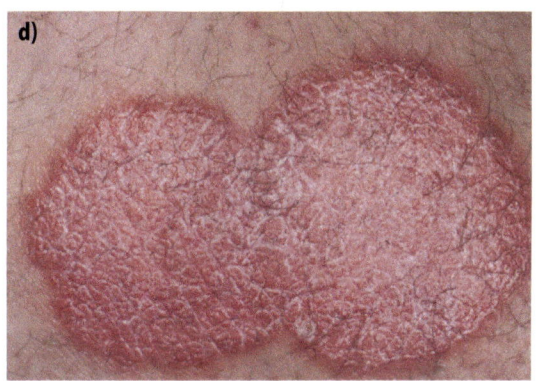

FIGURE 5.3. Plaque psoriasis lesions tend to be well demarcated with varying degrees of erythema, scale, and induration. **(a,b)** Depict thin plaques with minimal fine scale and erythema. **(c,d)** Show more indurated plaques with coarser scale that covers more of the lesion. **(e)** Depicts a plaque with beefy red erythema and coarse scaling that is often seen in untreated cases. **(f–h)** Show coarse, tenacious "silvery" scaling which are elevated 1–2 mm above normal skin.

(Continued)

Examples of plaque-type psoriasis

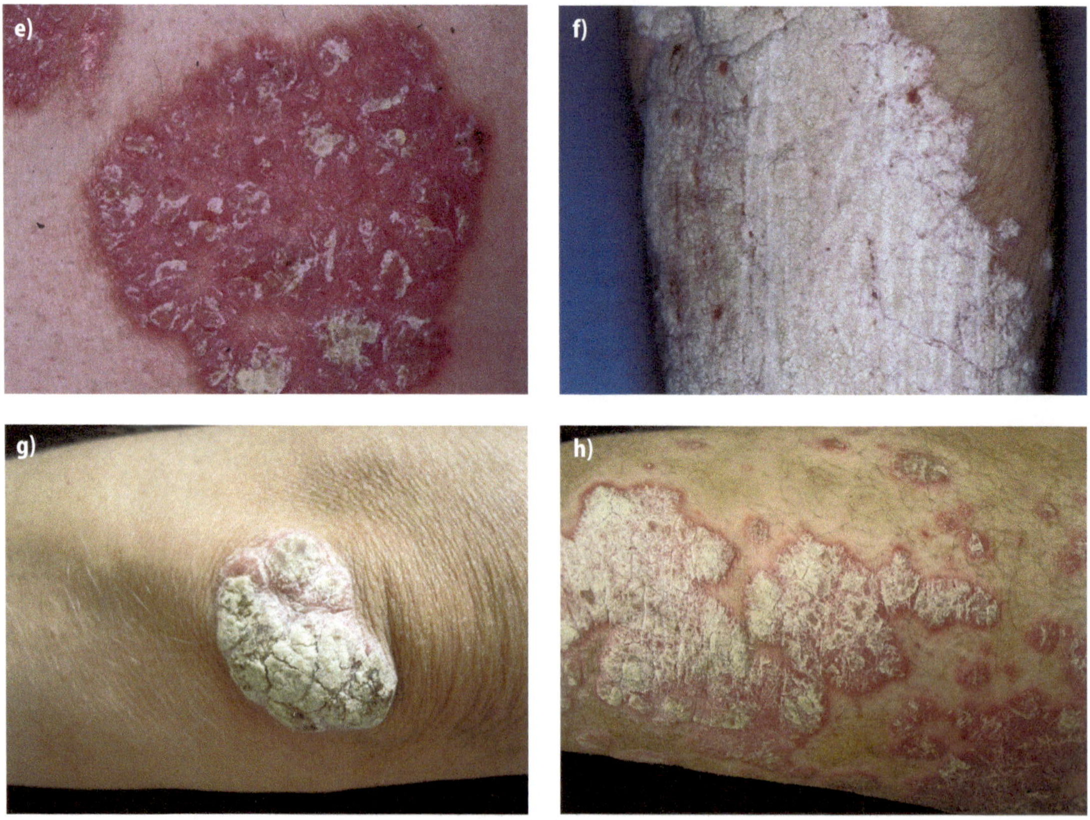

FIGURE 5.3. Continued

Examples of partially cleared psoriasis

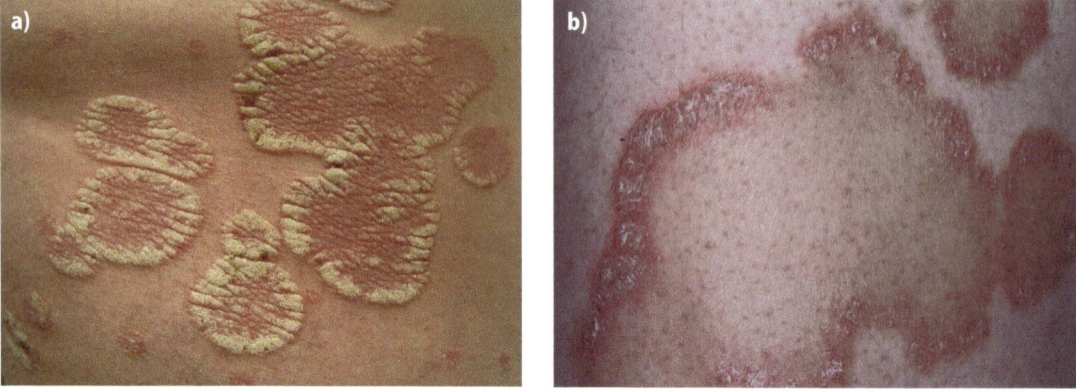

FIGURE 5.4. As psoriasis is treated, plaques may first clear centrally and take on an annular morphology (a,b) that can be mistaken for other dermatologic entities such as fungal infections or mycosis fungoides.

Guttate psoriasis

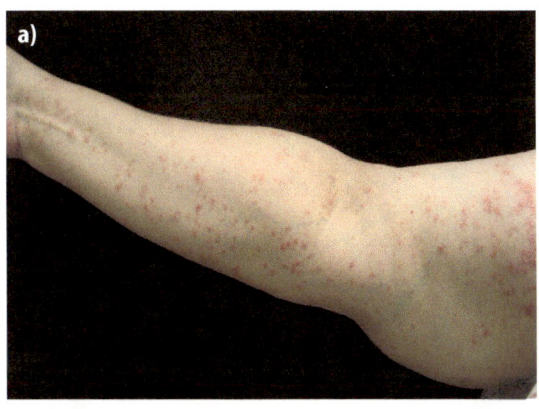

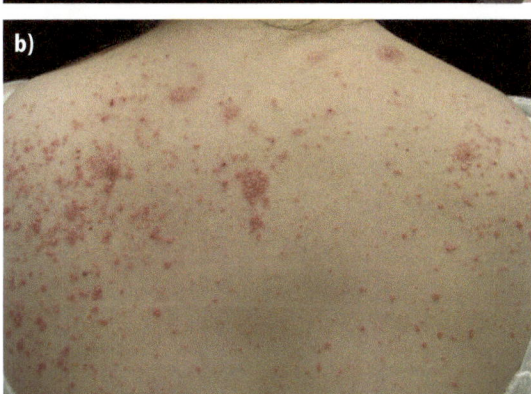

FIGURE 5.5. Guttate lesions **(a,b)** tend to be small scaly papules with bright red erythema and scale. Guttate psoriasis often presents in young adults and children following triggers including streptococcal pharyngitis, viral infections, medications, major stressors, or abrupt withdrawal of treatments (particularly corticosteroids or cyclosporine). Guttate psoriasis tends to respond well to topical agents and phototherapy.

Psoriatic flare

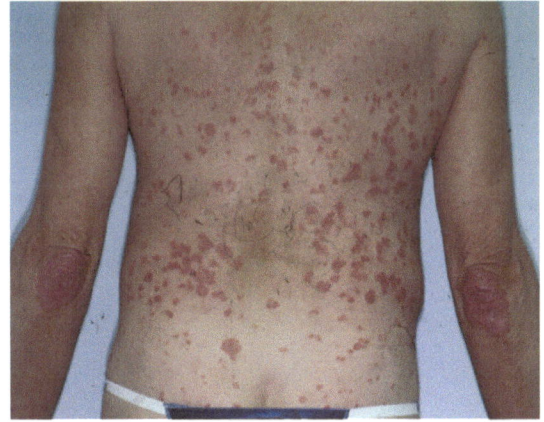

FIGURE 5.6. Patients with known plaque-type psoriasis may experience a flare with small plaques and guttate lesions.

Distribution of psoriasis

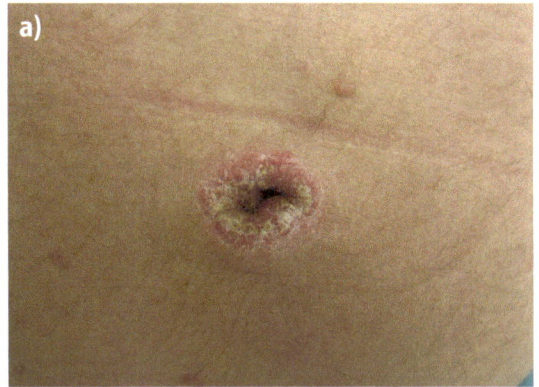

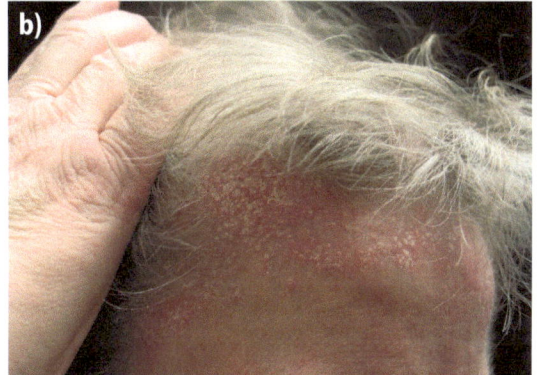

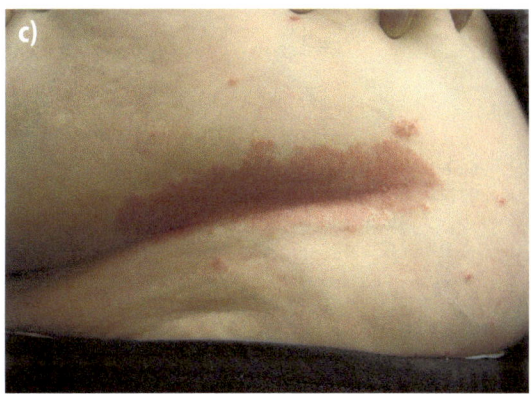

FIGURE 5.7. The distribution of plaques is often critical to making a diagnosis of psoriasis. The umbilicus **(a)** and scalp **(b)** are classically involved. Inverse psoriasis is defined as psoriasis in body folds **(c)**, axillae, and groin. It is often mistaken for intertrigo and fungal infections. Inverse lesions tend to be well-demarcated patches with minimal scale that tend to macerate and become secondarily infected with bacteria and yeast.

Palmoplantar psoriasis

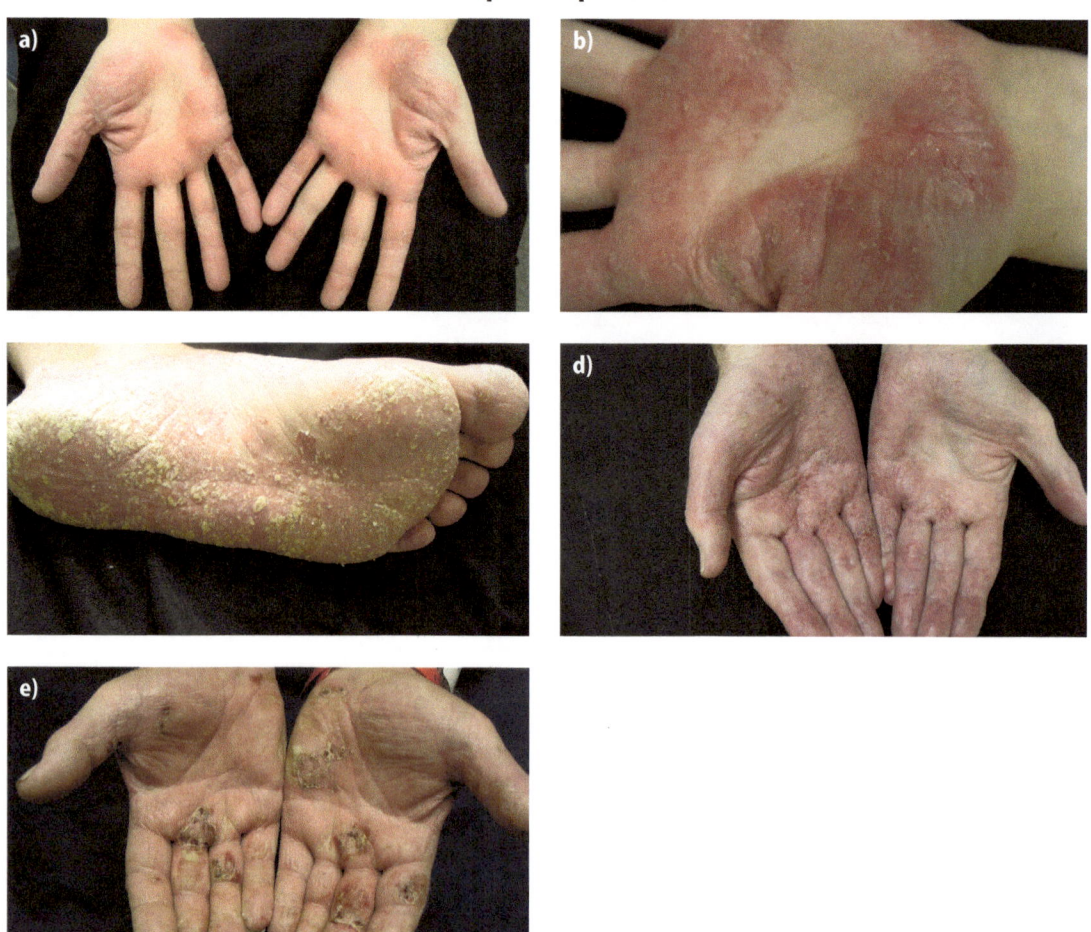

FIGURE 5.8. Psoriasis affecting the palms and soles, the palmo-plantar variant, has two variants: pustular and non-pustular. Non-pustular psoriasis **(a–c)** consists of typically well-demarcated hyperkeratotic plaques with scaling and fissuring, and can be difficult to differentiate from other disease such as hand eczema and contact dermatitis. Pustular palmoplantar disease is depicted in **(d)** and **(e)**. Palmoplantar disease, unlike other psoriasis variants such as guttate psoriasis, is not associated with the *PSORS1* susceptibility locus (HLA-C) [34]. Palmoplantar disease is difficult to treat with a topical regimen, and despite the limited body surface area involved, this disease can be very disabling and often requires systemic therapy, phototherapy, or photochemotherapy.

Erythrodermic psoriasis

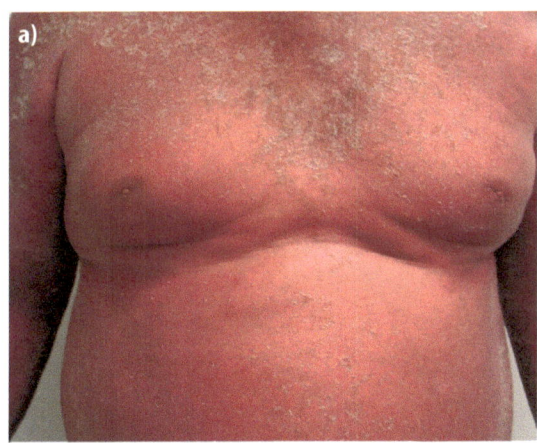 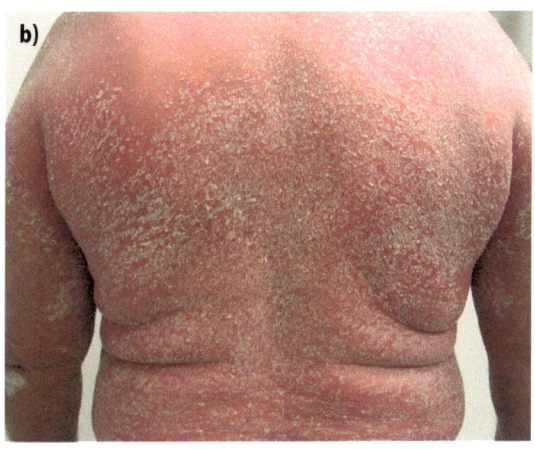

FIGURE 5.9. Erythrodermic psoriasis is a severe form of psoriasis characterized by widespread erythema, scaling, occasionally pustules (**a,b**), and often systemic illness including fever, hypotension, insensible fluid losses, and hypoalbuminemia. Erythrodermic psoriasis can be spontaneous but usually is associated with a trigger factor such as abrupt discontinuation of corticosteroids or other treatments, medications known to flare psoriasis such as lithium or β-blockers, and infection. Erythrodermic flares often require inpatient hospitalization in critical care units for management. It is important to differentiate from infection (sepsis) and other causes of erythroderma, such as Sézary syndrome, eczema, pytyriasis rubra pilaris, drug eruptions, and seborrheic dermatitis.

Pustular psoriasis

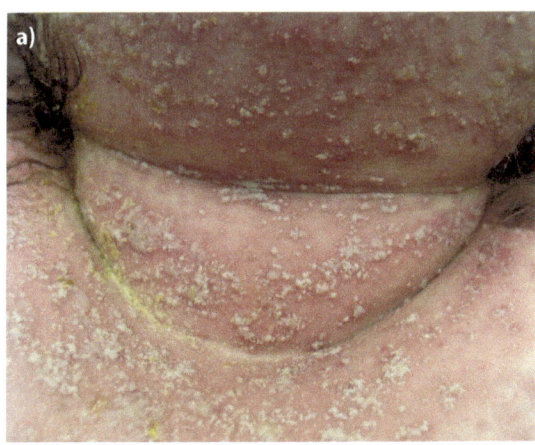 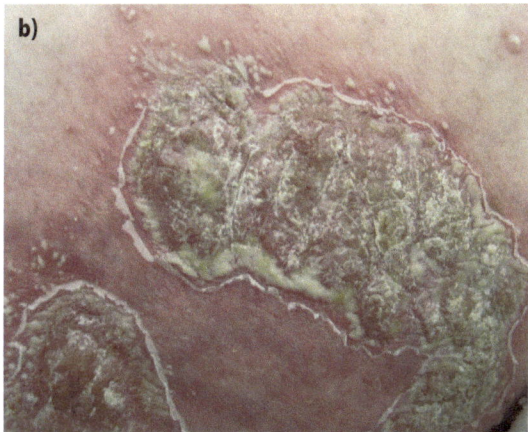

FIGURE 5.10. Pustular psoriasis (**a**) can occur as the primary form of psoriasis in an individual patient or in patients with established plaque-type psoriasis. Pustules usually develop after the rapid onset of erythema, rapidly, often with 'lakes of pus' forming at the edges of existing plaques (**b**). Acitretin (in patients not of childbearing potential) is usually the treatment of choice.

Psoriatic nail disease

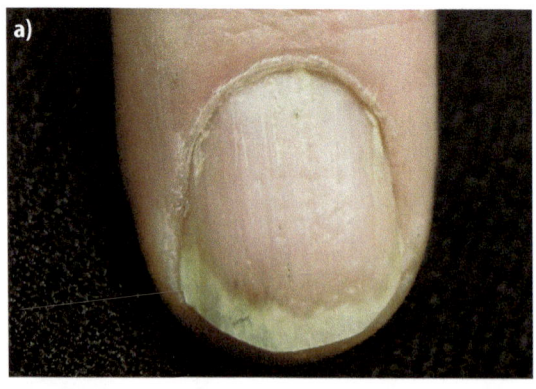
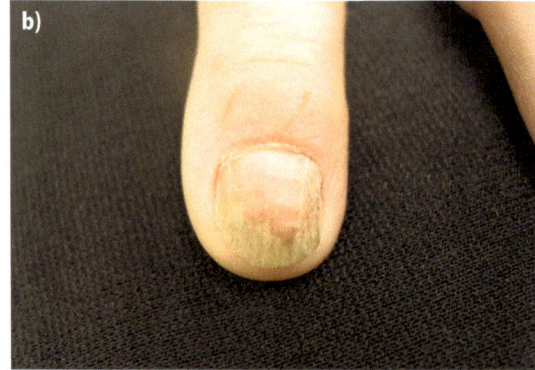
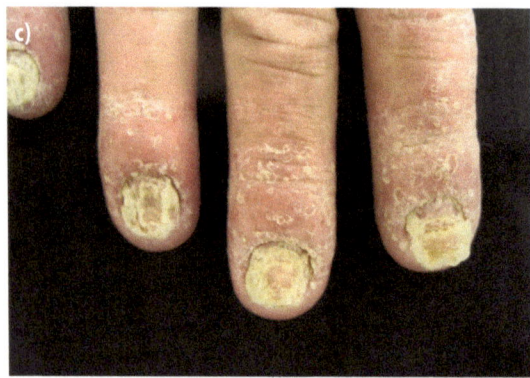
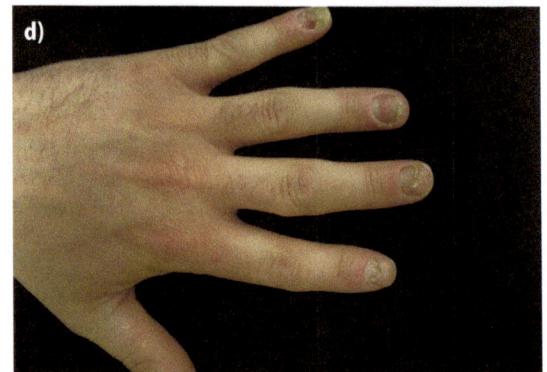

Figure 5.11. Psoriasis can involve both the fingernails and toenails, with the morphology ranging from minor abnormalities to disabling nail dystrophy. Characteristics of nail psoriasis include: pits, which are approximately 1-mm indentations that vary in number from nail to nail, best seen in (**a**); 'oil spots', or yellow-brown areas of discoloration, best seen in (**b**); and onycholysis (separation of the nail plate from the nail bed), subungal debris, and thickening and crumbling of the nail plate (**c**). Nails can be affected distally or proximally (**d**).

References

1. Krueger GG, Feldman SR, Camisa C *et al*. **Two considerations for patients with psoriasis and their clinicians: what defines mild, moderate, and severe psoriasis? What constitutes a clinically significant improvement when treating psoriasis?** *J Am Acad Dermatol* 2000; **43**(2, Pt 1):281–285.

2. Koo J. **Population-based epidemiologic study of psoriasis with emphasis on quality of life assessment.** *Dermatol Clin* 1996; **14**:485–496.

3. Henseler T, Christophers E. **Psoriasis of early and late onset: characterization of two types of psoriasis vulgaris.** *J Am Acad Dermatol* 1985; **13**:450–456.

4. Gudjonsson JE, Karason A, Antonsdottir AA *et al*. **HLA-Cw6-positive and HLA-Cw6-negative patients with Psoriasis vulgaris have distinct clinical features.** *J Invest Dermatol* 2002; **118**:362–365.

5. Banchereau J, Steinman RM. **Dendritic cells and the control of immunity.** *Nature* 1998; **392**:245–252.

6. Fuhlbrigge RC, Kieffer JD, Amerding D *et al*. **Cutaneous lymphocyte antigen is a specialized form of PSGL-1 expressed on skin-homing T cells.** *Nature* 1997; **389**:978–981.

7. Austin LM, Ozawa M, Kikuchi T *et al*. **The majority of epidermal T cells in psoriasis vulgaris lesions can produce type 1 cytokines, interferon-gamma, interleukin-2, and tumor necrosis factor-alpha, defining TC1 (cytotoxic T lymphocyte) and TH1 effector populations: a type 1 differentiation bias is also measured in circulating blood T cells in psoriatic patients.** *J Invest Dermatol* 1999; **113**:752–759.

8. Krueger JG. **The immunologic basis for the treatment of psoriasis with the new biologic agents.** *J Am Acad Dermatol* 2002; **46**:1–23.

9. Mehlis S, Gordon KB. **From laboratory to clinic: rationale for biologic therapy.** *Dermatol Clin* 2004; 22:371–377.

10. Drake LA, Ceilley RI, Cornelison RL *et al.* **Guidelines of care for psoriasis. Committee on Guidelines of Care. Task Force on Psoriasis.** *J Am Acad Dermatol* 1993; 28:632–637.

11. Biondi Oriente C, Scarpa R, Pucino A *et al.* **Psoriasis and psoriatic arthritis. Dermatological and rheumatological cooperative clinical report.** *Acta Derm Venereol Suppl* 1989; 146:69–71.

12. Boyd AS, Menter A. **Erythrodermic psoriasis. Precipitating factors, course, and prognosis in 50 patients.** *J Am Acad Dermatol* 1989; 21(5, Pt 1):985–991.

13. Gladman DD, Anhorn KA, Schachter RK *et al.* **HLA antigens in psoriatic arthritis.** *J Rheumatol* 1986; 13:586–592.

14. Elkayam O, Ophir J, Yaron M *et al.* **Psoriatic arthritis: interrelationships between skin and joint manifestations related to onset, course and distribution.** *Clin Rheumatol* 2000; 19:301–305.

15. Brandrup F, Holm N, Grunnet N *et al.* **Psoriasis in monozygotic twins: variations in expression in individuals with identical genetic constitution.** *Acta Derm Venereol* 1982; 62:229–236.

16. Swanbeck G, Inerot A, Martinsson T *et al.* **A population genetic study of psoriasis.** *Br J Dermatol* 1994; 131:32–39.

17. Abele DC, Dobson RL, Graham JB. **Heredity and psoriasis. Study of a large family.** *Arch Dermatol* 1963; 88:38–47.

18. Russell TJ, Schultes LM, Kuban DJ. **Histocompatibility (HL-A) antigens associated with psoriasis.** *N Engl J Med* 1972; 287:738–740.

19. Capon F, Trembath RC, Barker JN. **An update on the genetics of psoriasis.** *Dermatol Clin* 2004; 22:339–347.

20. Nair RP, Stuart P, Henseler T *et al.* **Localization of psoriasis-susceptibility locus PSORS1 to a 60-kb interval telomeric to HLA-C.** *Am J Hum Genet* 2000; 66:1833–1844.

21. Capon F, Munro M, Barker J *et al.* **Searching for the major histocompatibility complex psoriasis susceptibility gene.** *J Invest Dermatol* 2002; 118:745–751.

22. Asumalahti K, Veal C, Laitinen T *et al.* **Coding haplotype analysis supports HCR as the putative susceptibility gene for psoriasis at the MHC PSORS1 locus.** *Hum Mol Genet* 2002; 11:589–597.

23. Nair RP, Henseler T, Jenisch S *et al.* **Evidence for two psoriasis susceptibility loci (HLA and 17q) and two novel candidate regions (16q and 20p) by genome-wide scan.** *Hum Mol Genet* 1997; 6:1349–1356.

24. Trembath RC, Clough RL, Rosbotham JL *et al.* **Identification of a major susceptibility locus on chromosome 6p and evidence for further disease loci revealed by a two stage genome-wide search in psoriasis.** *Hum Mol Genet* 1997; 6:813–820.

25. Capon F, Semprini S, Dallapiccola B *et al.* **Evidence for interaction between psoriasis-susceptibility loci on chromosomes 6p21 and 1q21.** *Am J Hum Genet* 1999; 65:1798–1800.

26. Samuelsson L, Enlund F, Torinsson A *et al.* **A genome-wide search for genes predisposing to familial psoriasis by using a stratification approach.** *Hum Genet* 1999; 105:523–529.

27. Lee YA, Ruschendorf F, Windemuth C *et al.* **Genomewide scan in German families reveals evidence for a novel psoriasis-susceptibility locus on chromosome 19p13.** *Am J Hum Genet* 2000; 67:1020–1024.

28. Veal CD, Clough RL, Barber RC *et al.* **Identification of a novel psoriasis susceptibility locus at 1p and evidence of epistasis between PSORS1 and candidate loci.** *J Med Genet* 2001; 38:7–13.

29. Zhang XJ, He PP, Wang ZX *et al.* **Evidence for a major psoriasis susceptibility locus at 6p21 (PSORS1) and a novel candidate region at 4q31 by genome-wide scan in Chinese Hans.** *J Invest Dermatol* 2002; 119:1361–1366.

30. Helms C, Cao L, Krueger JG *et al.* **A putative RUNX1 binding site variant between SLC9A3 and NAT9 is associated with susceptibility to psoriasis.** *Nat Genet* 2003; 35:349–356.

31. Capon F, Helms C, Veal CD *et al.* **Genetic analysis of PSORS2 markers in a UK dataset supports the association between RAPTOR SNPs and familial psoriasis.** *J Med Genet* 2004; 41:459–460.

32. Matthews D, Fry L, Powles A *et al.* **Evidence that a locus for familial psoriasis maps to chromosome 4q.** *Nat Genet* 1996; 14:231–233.

33. Semprini S, Capon F, Tacconelli A *et al.* **Evidence for differential S100 gene over-expression in psoriatic patients from genetically heterogeneous pedigrees.** *Hum Genet* 2002; 111:310–313.

34. Asumalahti K, Ameen M, Suomela S *et al.* **Genetic analysis of PSORS1 distinguishes guttate psoriasis and palmoplantar pustulosis.** *J Invest Dermatol* 2003; 120:627–632.

6
Juvenile Psoriatic Arthritis

Helen Foster

Introduction

Musculoskeletal complaints in children are common, affecting 5–15% of children and adolescents [1]. The differential diagnosis is broad; in most cases the cause is mechanical rather than inflammatory in origin, often benign and self limiting, and without long-term sequelae. However, it must be remembered that some severe and even potentially life-threatening diseases can present with musculoskeletal symptoms and, therefore, it is always vital to consider and exclude conditions such as infection (septic arthritis or osteomyelitis), malignancy (leukemia, neuroblastoma, or bone tumor), severe trauma (including non-accidental injury), and some age-specific conditions that are unique to childhood (Perthes disease or slipped capital femoral epiphysis). Early and accurate diagnosis is important. A careful clinical history and examination, accompanied by knowledge of the normal musculoskeletal system in children and adolescents, and judicious use of a few appropriate investigations often leads to an accurate diagnosis.

Clinical Features of Juvenile Psoriatic Arthritis

Dactylitis

Single small joint involvement of the hand is typical of juvenile psoriatic arthritis (JPsA). Swelling of toes or fingers is known as dactylitis or 'sausage digit' and can be a good indicator of JPsA.

Psoriasis

The typical skin rash of psoriasis in children is similar to that of adults in the majority of cases; however, in children, the arthritis often appears several years before the rash, thus making JPsA very difficult to diagnose early on. As in adults, both genetic and environmental factors play a role in the development of psoriatic arthritis, and it is important to note whether there is a family history of psoriasis (as well as other forms of spondyloarthropathies).

Uveitis

The association of chronic anterior uveitis in juvenile idiopathic arthritis (JIA) is well described [2,3] and affects approximately 15–20% of children with JIA. The highest risk of uveitis in JIA is for girls in the preschool age group with oligoarticular disease, and who are antinuclear antibody positive and within 2 years of disease onset. In about 10% of cases uveitis can predate the onset of the arthritis, and as the onset of uveitis is usually insidious and often asymptomatic, this results in the delay in presentation and diagnosis. Undetected and untreated, visual loss can occur due to keratopathy, cataract, and glaucoma. In the early stages, uveitis may be only diagnosed by a slit lamp examination and regular ophthalmologic screening is recommended. Some children may report symptoms such as headache or change in vision, although the development of visual blurring suggests advanced uveitis and often a worse visual prognosis. In approximately two-thirds of cases, the changes can be bilateral.

The association of JPsA and uveitis is also well described and occurs in 15–20% of children with JPsA, often those who are antinuclear antibody positive. The uveitis in JPsA is similar to that of oligoarticular JIA, but there is a suggestion that this may be more resistant to topical steroids [2] and, furthermore, that boys may have more severe disease.

Growth Disturbances

Inflammatory joint disease can cause localized or generalized growth abnormalities [4]. Localized growth abnormalities cause increased or decreased bone growth depending on the site. The likely explanation is the differential effects of inflammatory hyperemia and altered weight bearing on the growth plates near the affected joints. Rapid growth occurs initially during active phases of the disease process, leading to a longer bone. It may subsequently lead to premature fusion of the epiphyses and, ultimately, relative shortening of the bone. Localized growth abnormalities are more common in late-presenting untreated disease, and are not uncommon in JPsA where the joint involvement is asymmetrical. Leg-length discrepancy occurring when knee arthritis of one leg causes more rapid leg growth, is more common in the younger child, can lead to functional disability, and ultimately a secondary scoliosis. Arthritis involving the foot and ankle or hand and wrist may result in a smaller foot or hand, respectively. In addition, temporomandibular joint disease can result in micrognathia [5].

Other Systemic Manifestations of JPsA

Most children with JPsA are not systemically unwell, but those with polyarthritis may present with malaise, lethargy, and even weight loss, fever, and poor growth. The acute-phase reactants are usually normal or mildly elevated. An uncommon but important syndrome to consider in the spectrum of JPsA presentation is that of chronic recurrent multifocal osteomyelitis (CRMO) [6], which is suggested to be the childhood equivalent of synovitis, acne, pustulosis, hyperostosis, and osteitis (SAPHO).

Imaging

The radiographic changes of JPsA are similar to that of JIA and may well be normal in early disease.

The changes within cartilage can take many months to appear and, consequently, radiographs are not routinely used to monitor disease activity or severity. Musculoskeletal ultrasound (MSUS) is increasingly used for imaging joints and periarticular changes.

Treatment

The management of JPsA is the same as that of JIA, with multidisciplinary care involving doctors, physiotherapists, occupational therapists, and nurses, in addition to close liaison with primary care and community healthcare services, as well as school and social services. The medical management focuses on earlier and more aggressive intervention based on evidence that joint damage occurs early and the poor long-term outcome for many patients. There is a paucity of evidence from clinical trials of immunosuppressive medication in JPsA, and the majority of pediatric rheumatologists, therefore, manage JPsA similar to the approach used in JIA. Most children are treated with non-steroidal anti-inflammatory drugs (NSAIDs) and intra-articular corticosteroids, and there is increasing use of methotrexate (MTX) and other forms of immunosuppressive regimes for polyarticular disease.

Outcome and Prognosis

There are few studies documenting the outcome of JPsA. However, it is generally regarded that, as a whole, these patients have a worse prognosis than most children with JIA. Polyarticular JPsA has a worse prognosis than oligoarticular JPsA. Follow-up studies suggest that two-thirds of patients have some functional limitation [7] and 10% have severe incapacity [8]. Long-term outcome studies demonstrate that quality of life for young adults with JIA is worse compared to their healthy peers, but there are no comparative studies of JPsA. These outcome studies reflect management trends from over a decade ago, which differ significantly from current approaches – the long-term impact of MTX and biologic therapies has yet to be determined.

Differential diagnosis of musculoskeletal disorders in children

Life-threatening conditions

- Malignancy (leukemia, lymphoma, bone tumor)
- Sepsis (septic arthritis, osteomyelitis)
- Non-accidental injury

Joint pain with no swelling

- Hypermobility syndromes
- Idiopathic pain syndromes (reflex sympathetic dystrophy, fibromyalgia)
- Orthopedic syndromes (eg, slipped capital femoral epiphysis, Osgood–Schlatter disease)
- Metabolic (eg, hypothyroidism)

Joint pain with swelling

- Juvenile idiopathic arthritis
- Trauma
- Infection
    - septic arthritis and osteomyelitis (viral, bacterial [including Lyme disease], mycobacterial)
    - reactive arthritis (post-enteric, sexually acquired)
    - infection related (rheumatic fever, vaccination related)
- Inflammatory bowel disease
- Connective tissue disease (systemic lupus erythematosus, scleroderma, dermatomyositis)
- Sarcoidosis
- Metabolic (eg, osteomalacia, cystic fibrosis)
- Hematological (hemophilia, hemoglobinopathy)
- Tumor (benign/malignant)
- Developmental/congenital (eg, spondylo-epiphyseal dysplasia)

FIGURE 6.1. When juvenile psoriatic arthritis (JPsA) is suspected, it is always vital to consider and exclude other conditions, especially life-threatening disorders that can also present with musculoskeletal symptoms.

Definition of JIA

Persistent arthritis >6 weeks

Age at onset under 16 years

Diagnosis of exclusion

FIGURE 6.2. The definition of arthritis is 'swelling within a joint or limitation in the range of movement of a joint *or* tenderness of a joint with limited range of movement'. The latter allows for the fact that swelling at some joints, such as the hip, temporomandibular joint, or subtalar joint, can be difficult to elicit clinically. These physical signs must be verified by a clinician and be present for a minimum of 6 weeks. Juvenile idiopathic arthritis (JIA) is a diagnosis of exclusion.

Comparison between the classification systems for JIA, JCA, and JRA

Characteristic	JIA	JRA	JCA
Age at onset (years)	<16	<16	<16
Minimum duration of arthritis	6 weeks	6 weeks	3 months
Subtypes			
Systemic	Arthritis, fever, rash	Systemic	Systemic
Oligoarthritis	1–4 joints affected during first 6–12 months	Pauciarticular JRA	Pauciarticular JCA
Persistent	Affects no more than 4 joints throughout course		
Extended	Affects >4 joints after first 6–12 months		
Polyarthritis			
RF⁻	Affects ≥5 joints first 6–12 months	Polyarticular JRA	Polyarticular JCA
RF⁺	Affects ≥5 joints first 6–12 months	Polyarticular JRA	JRA
Enthesitis-related arthritis*	Arthritis and enthesitis, or arthritis with at least two of following: sacroiliac tenderness, inflammatory back pain, HLA-B27⁺, family history of HLA-B27⁺-related disease	Excluded	Juvenile spondyloarthropathies
Psoriatic arthritis	*Arthritis and psoriasis, or arthritis with at least two of the following: dactylitis, nail changes, family history of psoriasis*		*Excluded*
Other	Arthritis of unknown cause or not fulfilling above categories		

FIGURE 6.3. The International League Against Rheumatism (ILAR) classification of JIA [9] is a consensus-derived classification system that replaces the former terms juvenile chronic arthritis (JCA) and juvenile rheumatoid arthritis (JRA), and is largely based on clinical features. This figure compares and contrasts the classification systems for JIA, JRA, and JCA. *Enthesitis is inflammation of the insertion of ligament, tendon, capsule, or fascia to bone, particularly around the foot and knee. RF, rheumatoid factor; HLA, human leukocyte antigen.

JIA and subtypes

Systemic

Polyarticular – RF⁻

Polyarticular – RF⁺

Oligoarticular

Extended oligoarthritis

Enthesitis-related/spondyloarthropathy

Psoriatic

Other

FIGURE 6.4. The term 'juvenile idiopathic arthritis', proposed by the ILAR classification [9], encompasses a heterogeneous group of conditions, reflected in the subtypes, which are essentially clinically, genetically, and serologically distinct from adult rheumatoid arthritis (RA). JPsA is one of these subtypes.

JPsA

ILAR criteria

Arthritis and psoriasis
OR
Arthritis and at least two of the following:

- dactylitis
- nail pitting or onycholysis
- family history of psoriasis in a first-degree relative

Vancouver criteria

Definite JPsA

- arthritis with typical psoriatic rash
OR
- arthritis with three of the following minor criteria:
  - nail pitting/psoriasis (first/second degree relative)
  - psoriasis-like rash
  - dactylitis

Probable JPsA

- arthritis with two/four minor criteria

FIGURE 6.5. Currently, two systems, which are not mutually exclusive, are used to classify the term JPsA and propose diagnostic criteria. The table lists the ILAR criteria [9] and also the Vancouver criteria [10]. One important feature of both the ILAR and Vancouver criteria is that a child can be diagnosed with JPsA without the classical rash of psoriasis; for example, a family history of psoriasis, or dactylitis in the absence of skin changes, will satisfy the definition of 'probable JPsA'. The reason for this is that for many children the arthritis may precede the psoriasis, and children with probable JPsA have a high risk of developing 'definite JPsA' with time [7], with a worse prognosis in terms of joint damage and of developing severe uveitis. It is important, therefore, to recognize this group of children early on and consider immunosuppressive medication to minimize joint damage and optimize outcome.

Guttate psoriasis

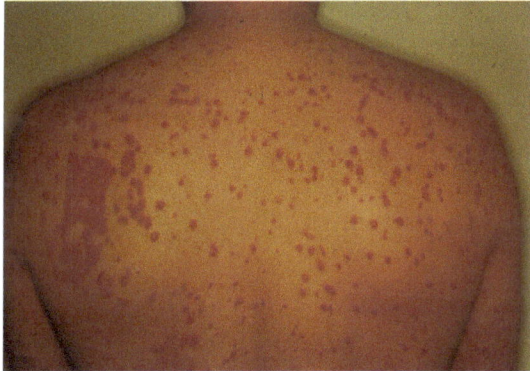

FIGURE 6.6. The cause of JIA and JPsA is unknown. There are case reports of psoriasis (and, in particular, guttate psoriasis) occurring after infections, such as streptococcal infections [11,12], although no association with JPsA and common viral infections has been observed [13]. Figure reproduced from *Atlas of Pediatrics* [14].

Epidemiology of JIA

a) Median age of onset and subtype of JIA

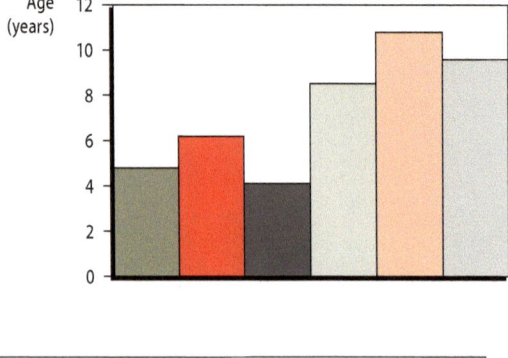

b) Relative incidence of JIA subtypes

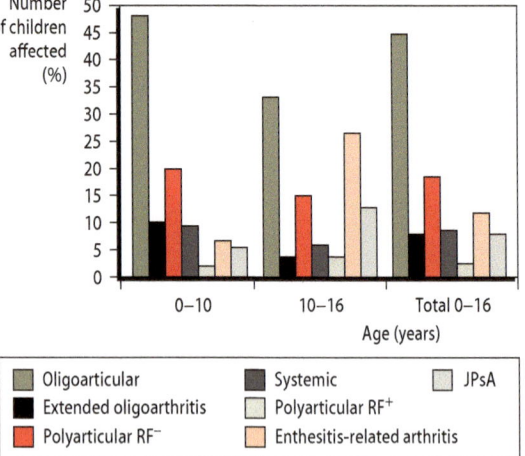

FIGURE 6.7. The incidence of chronic arthritis in childhood is approximately 1 in 10,000, with a prevalence of 1 in 1000 [3]. Oligoarticular JIA is the most common subtype at all ages, with a median age of onset of 4 years. JPsA accounts for 2–15% of children with chronic arthritis, with more recent studies stating approximately 7% [15,16]. Population studies suggest that the incidence of JPsA is 2.3–3 per 100,000 per year [17]. It is estimated that psoriasis affects 0.5% of young people under 16 years of age, which is much lower than in adults (approximately 1–3%). The proportion of patients with psoriasis who also have arthritis is unknown but may well be less than the 20–40% that is reported in adults. One of the problems in establishing incidence and prevalence is that, in contrast to adults with PsA where the rash often precedes the arthritis by several years, in children the opposite is true (ie, the arthritis often precedes the rash). This may explain the reported earlier age of onset of probable JPsA (7 ± 4.5 years) compared to definite JPsA (10 ± 4.9 years) [18]. There are few studies of ethnic association and JPsA, but one multicenter survey of patients with definite JPsA in the USA demonstrated a predominance of patients being White (>90%), with 5% being Hispanic and 2.5% being African-American [19]. The gender ratio is almost equal males to females, which is unusual for JIA as a whole, as it predominantly affects girls. The peak age of onset of JPsA is in middle-to-late childhood (approximately 10 years of age), although a lesser peak appears to be in the pre-school age group, and mostly in girls [10].

Clinical features of JPsA

	Lambert [19]	Calabro [20]	Sills [21]	Shore & Ansell [8]	Wesolowska [22]	Southwood [10]	Total
Year	1976	1977	1980	1980	1995	1989	–
Patients (n)	43	12	24	60	21	35	195
Male / female ratio	11:32	5:7	7:17	35:25	13:8	23:11	0.95:1
Age at onset of joint disease (years)	9.3	NA	10	11	NA	6.7	6.7–11.0
Age at onset of skin disease (years)	10.4	NA	11	8.8	NA	12.6	8.8–12.6
Disease sequence							
psoriasis first (%)	40	67	33	42	33	43	33–67
arthritis first (%)	53	33	58	43	62	48	33–62
simultaneous (%)	7	0	9	15	5	10	5–15
Oligoarticular onset (%)	55	42	58	73	86	94	42–94
Polyarticular onset (%)	45	58	42	27	14	6	6–58
DIP joints affected (%)	21	50	62	42	10	29	10–62
Sacroiliac changes (%)	28	17	29	47*	100*	11	11–100
Nail changes (%)	70	92	83	77	86	51	51–92
Uveitis (%)	9	0	13	8	14	17	0–17

FIGURE 6.8. *Selected patients had pelvic radiographs. Summary of reported series adapted from *Textbook of Paediatric Rheumatology* [23].

FIGURE 6.9. **(a)** Shows JPsA patterns of joint disease at onset. The most common rheumatologic presentation of JIA is oligoarticular disease and the knee is the most frequently affected joint at initial presentation. In JPsA, an oligoarticular onset is also most common (70% of cases) with other forms being less common [7]. Other forms of the disease, such as asymmetrical polyarthritis or distal interphalangeal (DIP) joint disease with nail changes, are observed as in adult-onset PsA, but are much less common in children. Sacroiliitis involvement is unusual in children with JPsA but often associates with HLA-B27 positivity; in some cases where enthesitis is also a feature, these children may be classified as the enthesitis-related arthritis subtype of JIA. This clearly highlights one of the difficulties in the proposed ILAR classification. An oligoarticular onset of joint disease is most common in JPsA; in one study of 63 children with JPsA, 73% of children have an oligoarticular onset, and even in those with a polyarticular onset, the median number of joints involved at onset was only 6 (range 5–10) [7]. However, there is a tendency for children with JPsA to have cumulative joint involvement **(b)**, and many children who present with oligoarticular disease progress to polyarticular involvement and a more guarded prognosis [7,8,24]. MCP, metacarpophalangeal; MTP, metatarsophalangeal.

a) JPsA patterns of joint disease at onset

Oligoarthritis (<5 joints)	70%
Symmetrical polyarthritis (≥5 joints)	15%
Predominant DIP joints	5%
Sacroiliitis with peripheral arthritis	5%
Arthritis mutilans	5%

b) Joint involvement in JPsA

	Onset (%)	Cumulative (%)
Knee	50	80
Finger	25	50
Toe	25	45
Ankle	29	60
Wrist	10	10
Elbow	10	30
Hindfoot	5	30
MCP	5	50
DIP (finger)	5	40
MTP	5	30
Cervical spine	5	30
Sacroiliac joints	2	5
Hip	5	25
Strenoclavicular	2	10
Temporomandibular	1	30
Shoulder	1	10

Oligoarticular-onset JPsA

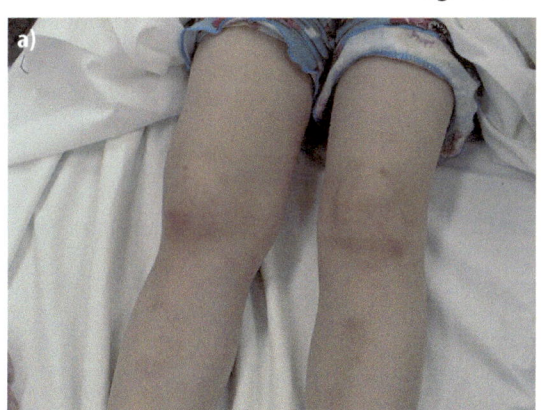 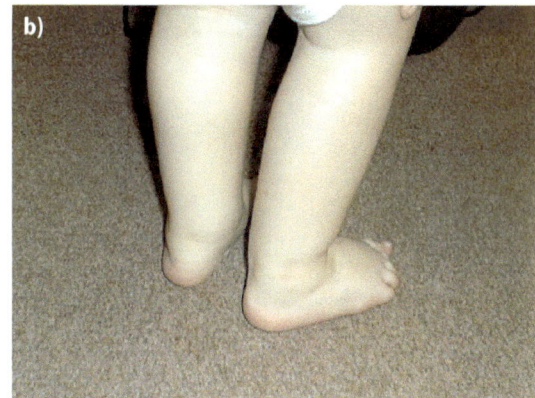

FIGURE 6.10. **(a)** Oligoarticular-onset JPsA affecting the right knee. **(b)** Oligoarticular-onset JPsA with involvement of the ankles. The swelling of the ankles may be more obvious from inspection of the child from behind.

Asymmetrical small joint involvement in JPsA

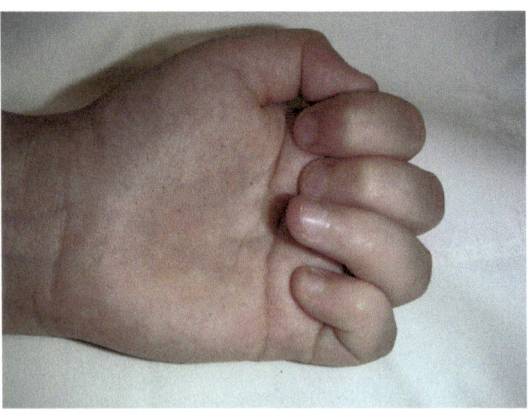 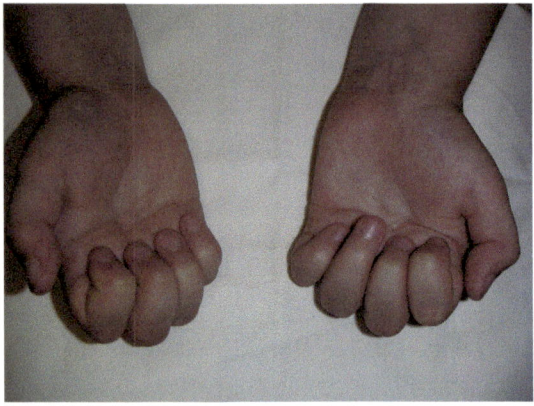

FIGURE 6.11. JPsA with asymmetrical joint involvement of the fingers. Note the inability to fully flex the left ring finger DIP joint in a child with JPsA.

Symmetrical DIP involvement in JPsA

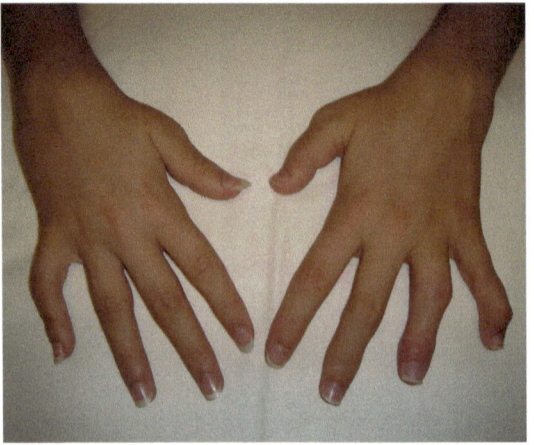

FIGURE 6.12. Symmetrical DIP joint involvement in JPsA is often associated with nail changes (*see* Figure 6.27).

Polyarticular JPsA

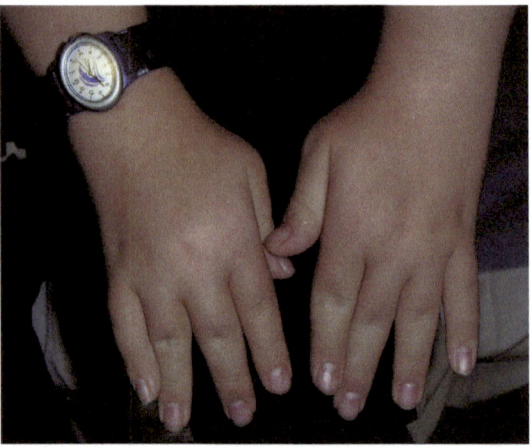

FIGURE 6.13. Polyarticular JPsA involving MCP joints and proximal interphalangeal (PIP) joints in the hands, as well as both wrists.

Psoriasis skin rash

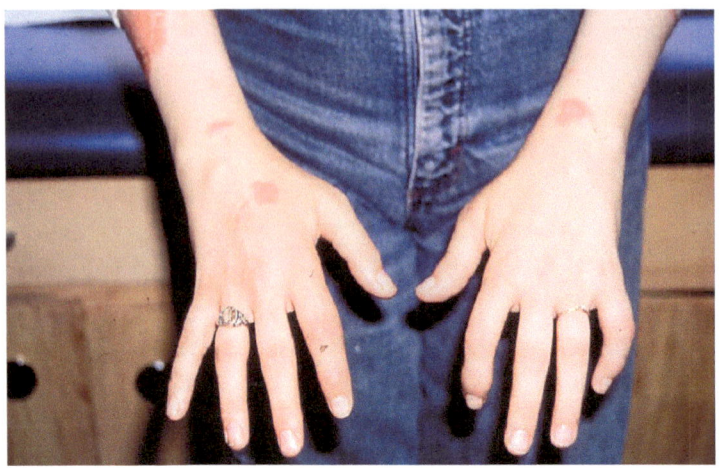

FIGURE 6.14. Asymmetrical small joint disease of the hands in association with psoriasis skin rash is typical of JPsA. Photo courtesy of Dr Mark Friswell, Newcastle Hospitals NHS Trust.

Destructive small joint disease in JPsA

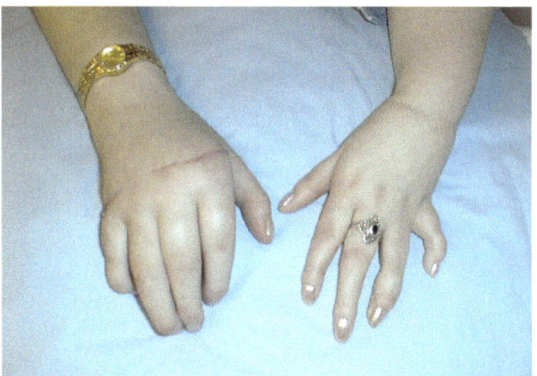

FIGURE 6.15. Asymmetrical destructive small joint disease involving MCP, PIP and DIP joints in a young adult with JPsA. Note the scars of small joint surgery.

Oligoarticular-onset JIA or oligoarticular JPsA?

Small joint involvement (hands/feet)

Wrist involvement

Dactylitis

Family history of psoriasis

FIGURE 6.16. The skin rash of psoriasis may not appear in JPsA until many years after the onset of arthritis [10]. It is often, therefore, difficult to distinguish between JIA and JPsA, particularly as an oligoarticular presentation is most common in both subtypes. However, the prognosis for JPsA is generally regarded as much worse than oligoarticular JIA, and making an accurate diagnosis is important in planning management and counseling the family.

This figure shows the key features that are suggestive of JPsA in the early stages of the disease course, especially when the child does not have psoriasis. Such indicative features include involvement, especially asymmetrically, of small joint(s) of a digit in the hand or foot, wrist disease, dactylitis, and/or a family history of a relative with psoriasis or psoriatic arthritis [24]. A retrospective study compared the clinical features and patterns of joint involvement of children with oligoarticular JIA and oligoarticular JPsA [24]: the presence of small joint disease of the hand or foot (defined as involvement of any of the MTP, PIP or DIP joints of the foot, or MCP, PIP or DIP joints of the hand) was significantly more frequent in oligoarticular JPsA than in oligoarticular JIA at disease onset. The odds of patients with oligoarticular JPsA having small joint disease or wrist disease within 6 months of disease onset were much higher than those with oligoarticular JIA ($p < 0.05$ or $p < 0.001$) [24].

Knee arthritis and asymmetrical growth

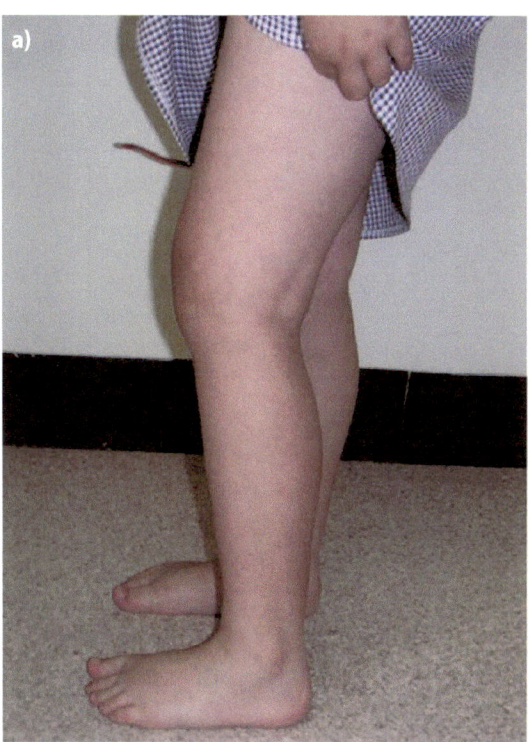

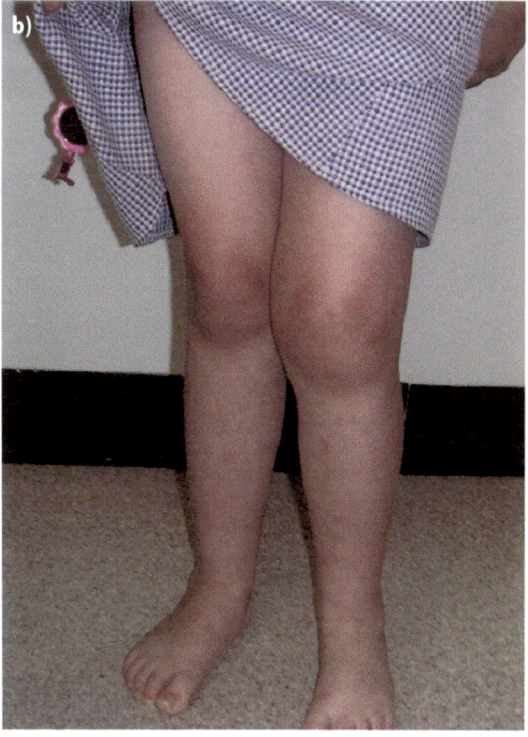

FIGURE 6.17. Flexion contracture and leg-length overgrowth at the left knee with oligoarticular-onset JPsA. Leg-length discrepancy, occurring when knee arthritis of one leg causes more rapid leg growth, is more common in the younger child, can lead to functional disability, and ultimately can cause a secondary scoliosis.

JPsA of the left foot and asymmetrical growth

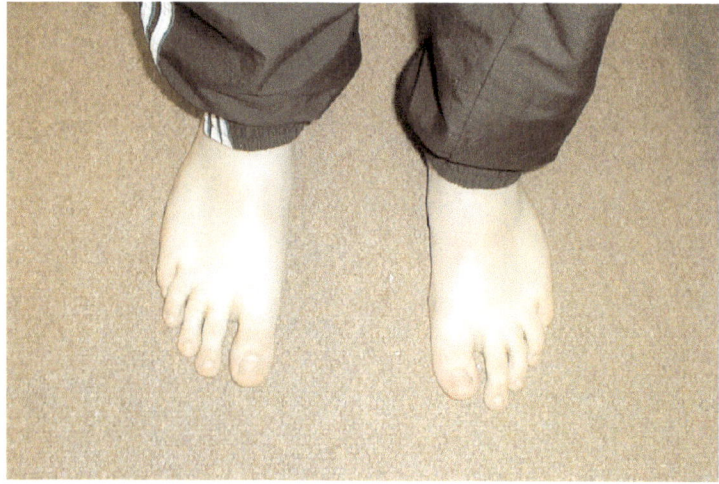

FIGURE 6.18. JPsA affecting first MTP and interphalangeal joint in the left foot resulting in asymmetrical growth, and leading to a shortened left great toe.

Micrognathia

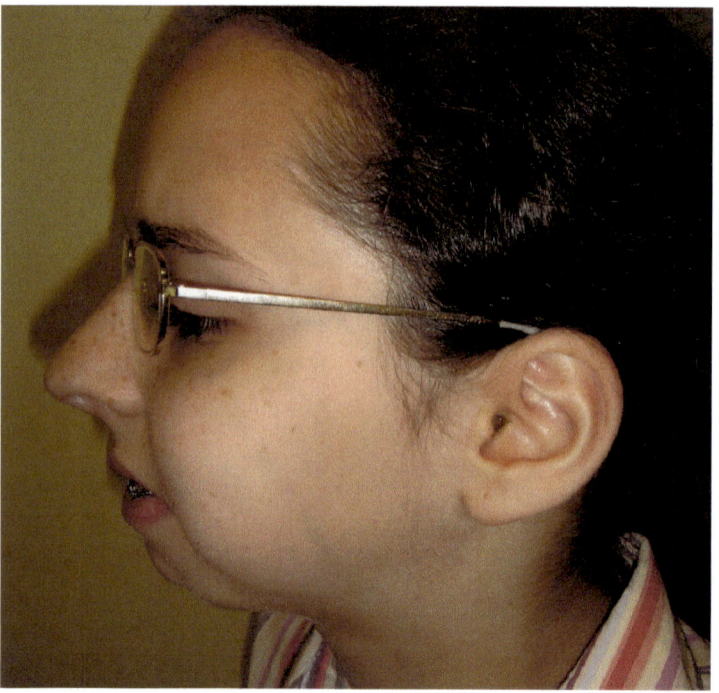

FIGURE 6.19. Temporomandibular joint disease can result in micrognathia (due to decreased and abnormal growth of the jaw) with or without jaw deviation. This creates difficulties in eating, speaking and toothbrushing, which can result in poor oral health and caries [5]. There may also be a considerable cosmetic impact.

Dactylitis

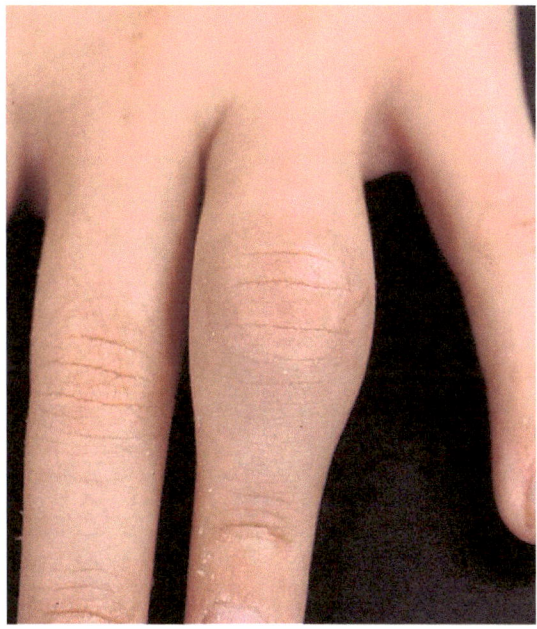

FIGURE 6.20. Dactylitis, or 'sausage digit', results from the combined inflammation of joint and tendons and affects the fingers and toes. The swelling extends beyond the joint (ie, it is periarticular), and is often in isolation from arthritis elsewhere and, thus, may be easily overlooked. One series reports dactylitis being present in 49% of patients with JPsA [10].

The differential diagnosis of dactylitis must include sepsis, foreign body synovitis, and tumor.

Dactylitis in the foot

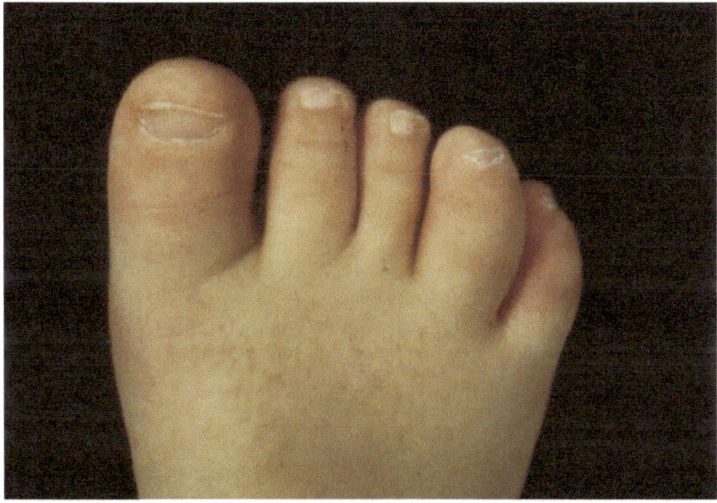

FIGURE 6.21. Note the swelling of the whole digit of the right fourth toe and the onycholysis in the nails of the adjacent toes, suggestive of psoriasis.

Case history: dactylitis in the left foot

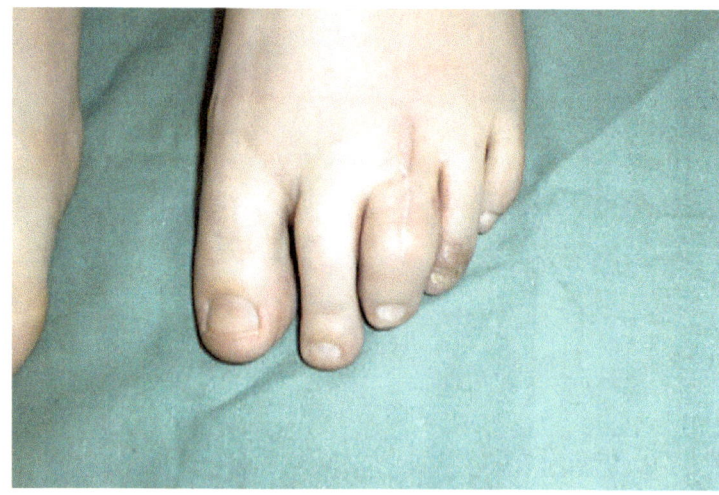

FIGURE 6.22. Note the surgical scar along the dorsum of the third toe. This 8-year-old child presented with a swollen toe. He was, however, feeling well, apyrexial, and with no history of trauma. Investigations revealed a normal full blood count and normal acute-phase reactants. There was no family history of note and, in particular, no history of psoriasis. He was initially investigated for presumed septic arthritis and osteomyelitis. The toe was surgically explored; the synovial biopsy was sterile, but revealed non-specific chronic inflammatory changes. There was no response to antibiot- ics. After 6 months, he was referred to pediatric rheumatology for the first time. At this stage he had no joint symptoms of note but physical examination revealed lack of full extension at his elbow, swelling and limited movement of the DIP joint of his right middle finger, in addition to the dactylitis and changes of psoriasis in the fourth toe adjacent to the dactylitis. The diagnosis was JPsA and this case history illustrates a typical case presentation with delay to diagnosis and pediatric rheumatology care – a scenario that is not uncommon.

Enthesitis

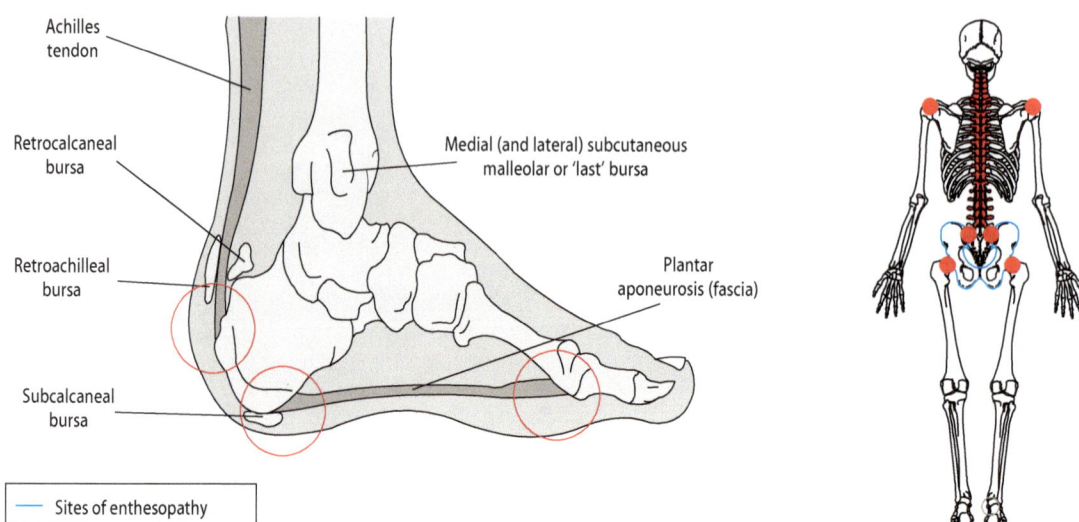

FIGURE 6.23. Enthesitis is the site of attachment of tendon, liga- ment, fascia, or capsule to bone. It is reported to be a cardinal feature of adult-onset psoriatic arthritis [25] and classically occurs at the foot and heel. Although enthesis can be observed in chil- dren with psoriasis, it is invariably associated with being HLA-B27 positive and the clinical features are more typical of the enthesitis- related arthritis subtype of JIA.

Heel and foot pain in children

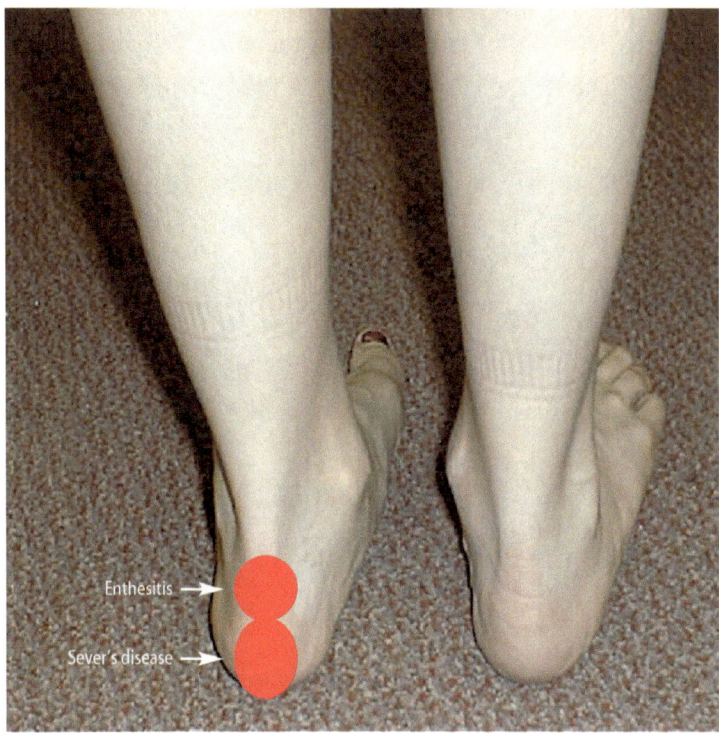

FIGURE 6.24. Heel and foot pain are common presenting musculoskeletal complaints in children and adolescents. Enthesitis, although uncommon, must be considered in the differential diagnosis. In the majority of cases, trauma, ill-fitting shoes, and localized soft tissue causes (eg, verrucae, foreign body) are likely alternative causes. The characteristic feature of enthesitis, however, is exquisite and localized tenderness at the enthesis, as opposed to tenderness over the calcaneum itself, which is more typical of Sever's disease (a form of osteochondritis, often related to physical activity and not a feature of JIA).

Psoriasis at the umbilicus

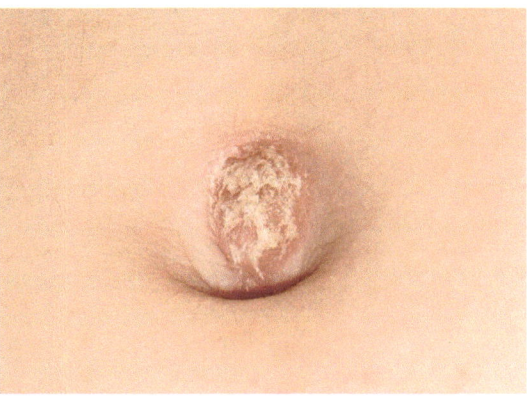

FIGURE 6.25. The typical skin rash of psoriasis in children is similar to that of adults in the majority of cases, with scaly erythematous patches over the extensor surfaces of the elbows and knees. However, in contrast to adult psoriatic arthritis, juvenile arthritis often precedes the rash by several years, and a high index of suspicion is required in the presence of arthritis of the small joints of the hands, feet and wrists, asymmetrical large and small joint disease, and dactylitis. Careful history taking should include enquiry about 'dandruff' to suggest scalp involvement or a family history of psoriasis. Careful examination should note any features of rash, especially around the umbilicus, behind the ears, and natal cleft.

Less common forms of skin rash in children include guttate psoriasis (*see* Figure 6.6), pustular psoriasis, and even erythrodermic psoriasis. Copyright of The Newcastle Upon Tyne Hospitals NHS Trust.

Koebner phenomenon

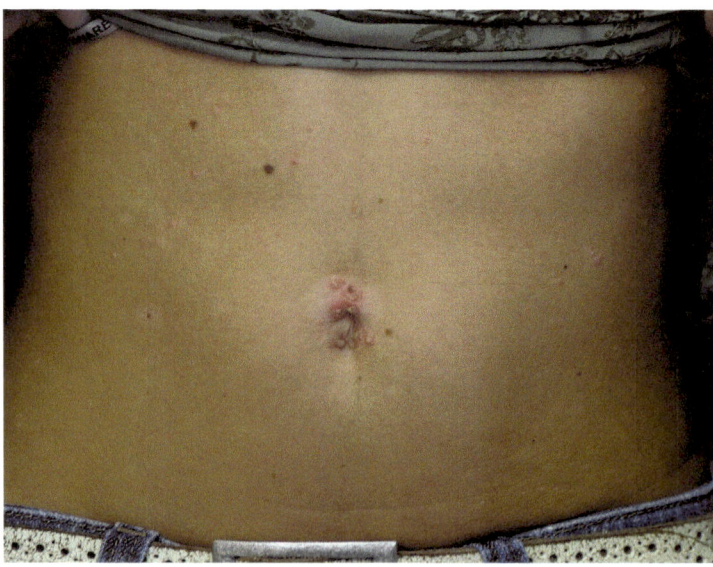

FIGURE 6.26. A Koebner phenomenon – where psoriasis occurs at sites of skin trauma – is recognized in psoriatic arthritis in both adults and children. This figure demonstrates Koebner phenome-non following naval piercing; note the small plaque psoriatic lesions elsewhere on the abdomen. Photo courtesy of Dr Lesley Kay, Newcastle University.

Nail changes

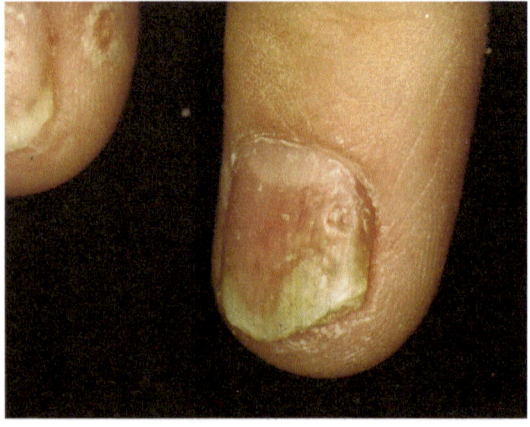

FIGURE 6.27. Nail pitting may be subtle and must be carefully looked for, as this may be the only feature of psoriasis in the child and therefore helpful for diagnosis and prognosis. Other features of nail involvement in JPsA are less common and include ony-cholysis, dystrophy, and horizontal ridging. Nail changes in JPsA are often associated with DIP joint involvement, and it is suggested that the nail changes are due to enthesitis at the nail bed [25].

Acute anterior uveitis

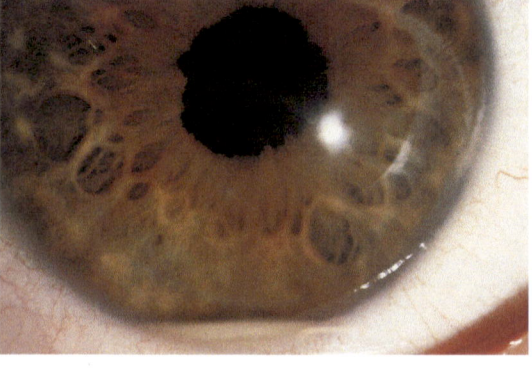

FIGURE 6.28. Acute anterior uveitis (ie, a painful red eye) is less common in JIA and is associated with enthesitis-related arthritis and being HLA-B27 positive. Children with enthesitis-related arthritis are therefore more at risk of acute anterior uveitis rather than chronic anterior uveitis. Note the injected eye with hypopyon in the anterior chamber.

FIGURE 6.29. Chronic anterior uveitis is described as an inflammatory disease of the anterior part of the eye lasting for more than 3 months. JIA-associated uveitis is linked with significant ocular morbidity and is the most common cause of chronic anterior uveitis in childhood. Complications of uveitis include cataract, glaucoma, keratopathy, and permanent visual loss. Approximately 10% of children with JPsA also develop uveitis. In the early stages, the eyes looks normal and uveitis can only be detected by slit lamp examination. Late-stage uveitis results in visual loss from keratopathy, glaucoma, and cataract.

Chronic anterior uveitis

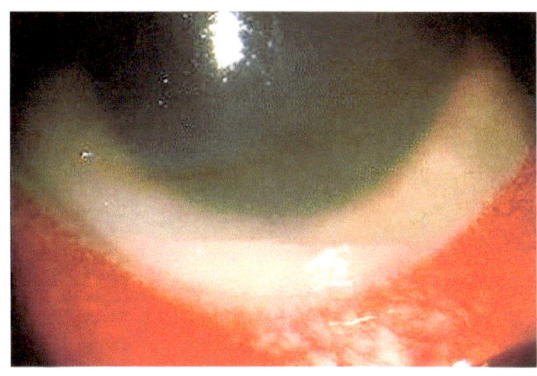

Recommended ophthalmologic monitoring for patients with JIA

Risk	Interval for screening (months)	Presence of antinuclear antibody	Subtype of JIA	Age at onset	Disease duration
Low	12	–	Systemic	Any	–
		+ or –	Polyarticular	Any	>7 years
Moderate	6	+ or –	Polyarticular	<7 years	–
		–	Oligoarticular	<7 years	<8 years
		+	Oligoarticular	<7 years	>7 years
High	3–4	+	Oligoarticular	<7 years	<8 years

FIGURE 6.30. The changes in the early stages can only be detected by a slit lamp examination by a skilled ophthalmologist. Regular screening is strongly advocated and the frequency of screening is influenced by the level of risk. In the UK, the British Society for Paediatric and Adolescent Rheumatology advocate regular screening for at least 5 years or until the child reaches 12 years [26], although these guidelines are currently under revision. Figure reproduced from Cassidy et al [23].

MSUS image of an adolescent with JPsA

FIGURE 6.31. Musculoskeletal ultrasound (MSUS) may be more readily available than magnetic resonance imaging, is sensitive to early changes of synovitis and enthesitis, well tolerated in children, portable, and can be used in a dynamic setting [27]. It, therefore, has enormous potential use in children, particularly as radiographs are often normal in early disease (as the joints are predominantly cartilaginous). This figure shows an MSUS image of an MCP joint in an adolescent with JPsA, and demonstrates active synovitis, enthesitis, and erosive changes.

The use of MSUS and Power Doppler have been reported in JIA [28,29], but there are no published reports of MSUS in JPsA. Photo courtesy of Dr David Kane and Dr Jo Cunington, Newcastle University.

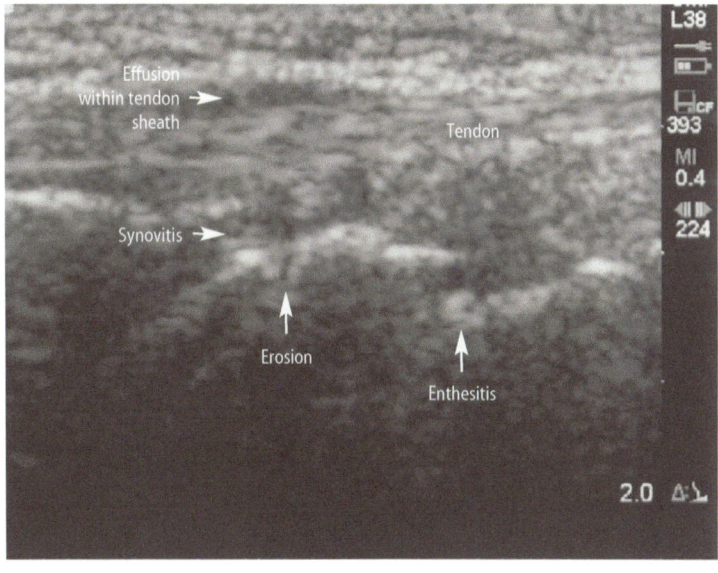

Medicines used to treat inflammatory arthritis in children

Non-steroidal anti-inflammatory drugs (NSAIDs)

	Daily dose (mg/kg/day)
Ibuprofen	20–40
Naproxen	10–15
Piroxicam	10–20
Diclofenac	2–3
Indomethacin	1–2

Notes:
- combinations of NSAIDs are not used
- salicylates are not recommended because of the risk of Reye's syndrome
- indomethacin slow-release preparations are often given at night to reduce morning stiffness
- sugar-free syrups should be prescribed wherever possible to reduce the risk of dental caries
- there is no licence currently available for cyclooxygenase (COX)-2-selective inhibitors to be used in children

Corticosteroids

	Dose for intra-articular use (mg/kg)
Triamcinolone hexa/acetonide	1–2 large joints (eg, knee)
Prednisolone acetate	10–20 small joints (eg, MCPs)

Disease-modifying antirheumatic drugs (DMARDs)

Methotrexate

Sulfasalazine

Leflunamide

(Cyclosporine)

Biologics and anticytokine therapies

Etanercept (only anti-TNF-α medication licensed for use in JIA)

Infliximab

Adalimumab

FIGURE 6.32. The main objectives of treatment are to help the child maintain a normal level of physical and social activity and optimize quality of life. Management is by a multidisciplinary team and will include medication and physical therapy (either with a physiotherapist or an occupational therapist) to achieve these goals.

The exposure to oral corticosteroids is minimized with increasing use of intra-articular corticosteroids (triamcinolone hexacetonide/acetonide) and early use of DMARDs, especially MTX. Pulsed intravenous methylprednisolone is used for severe polyarthritis and is a useful bridging agent when starting MTX therapy. Daily calcium and vitamin D supplements are often given to reduce the risk of osteoporosis. Topical corticosteroids are used to treat uveitis, although MTX (or tacrolimus) is also useful. NSAIDs are commonly used with sugar-free preparations being advocated to miminize caries risk. MTX is widely used, is efficacious [30] and well tolerated with few side effects. There are very few reports of serious complications (eg, liver fibrosis, pneumonitis), and the theoretical risks of malignancy and infertility have not been reported. MTX given by a subcutaneous route improves bioavailability and tolerability [31]. Alternative DMARD therapy (eg, leflunamide, cyclosporine, sulfasalazine) may be given as single agents or in combination therapy with MTX, but there is considerable toxicity and poor evidence of efficacy. The drugs gold and penicillamine and hydroxychloroquine are very rarely used due to poor efficacy and considerable toxicity [32]. Intra-articular corticosteroid is highly effective and safe [33], with triamcinolone hexacetonide being more efficacious than triamcinolone acetonide [34]. Early use of intra-articular corticosteroid in oligoarticular JIA and oligoarticular JPsA is advocated – in the case of knee involvement, the earlier the joint injection in the course of the disease, the less risk there is of leg-length discrepancy and muscle wasting [35]. Ultrasound imaging is increasingly used to facilitate accurate injection and especially to relatively inaccessible joints (eg, subtalar and hip joints).

Etanercept (a soluble tumor necrosis factor (TNF)-α receptor fusion protein) is the sole agent currently with a licence for use in refractory polyarticular JIA (and including JPsA if there is polyarticular involvement). In the UK, there are stringent criteria for use [36], and monitoring (for safety and efficacy) is mandatory (*www.bspar.org.uk*). Evidence to date, shows dramatic and sustained improvement with reduced joint damage in approximately two-thirds of patients with JIA [37,38]. It is likely that further anti-cytokine agents will be licensed for use in JIA in the future, following very promising evidence of their use in adults with RA and psoriatic arthritis.

References

1. Goodman JE, McGrath PJ. **The epidemiology of pain in children and adolescents – a review.** *Pain* 1991; 46:247–264.

2. Cabral DA, Petty RE, Malleson PN *et al.* **Visual prognosis in children with chronic anterior uveitis and arthritis.** *J Rheumatol* 1994; 21:2370–2375.

3. Rosenberg AM. **Uveitis associated with juvenile rheumatoid arthritis.** *Semin Arthritis Rheum* 1987; 16:158–173.

4. White PH. **Growth abnormalities in children with juvenile rheumatoid arthritis.** *Clin Orthop Relat Res* 1990; 259:46–50.

5. Welbury RR, Thomason JM, Fitzgerald LJ *et al.* **Increased prevalence of dental caries and poor oral hygiene in juvenile idiopathic arthritis.** *Rheumatology* 2003; 42:1445–1451.

6. Laxer RM, Shore AD, Manson D *et al.* **Chronic recurrent multifocal osteomyelitis and psoriasis – a report of a new association and review of related disorders.** *Semin Arthritis Rheum* 1988; 17:260–270.

7. Roberton DM, Cabral DA, Malleson PN *et al.* **Juvenile psoriatic arthritis: followup and evaluation of diagnostic criteria.** *J Rheumatol* 1996; 23:166–170.

8. Shore A, Ansell BM. **Juvenile psoriatic arthritis – an analysis of 60 cases.** *J Pediatr* 1982; 100:529–535.

9. Petty RE. **Growing pains: the ILAR classification of juvenile idiopathic arthritis.** *J Rheumatol* 2001; 28:927–928.

10. Southwood TR, Petty RE, Malleson PN *et al.* **Psoriatic arthritis in children.** *Arthritis Rheum* 1989; 32:1007–1013.

11. Vasey FB, Deitz C, Fenske NA *et al.* **Possible involvement of group A streptococci in the pathogenesis of psoriatic arthritis.** *J Rheumatol* 1982; 9:719–722.

12. Telfer NR, Chalmers RJ, Whale K *et al.* **The role of streptococcal infection in the initiation of guttate psoriasis.** *Arch Dermatol* 1992; 128:39–42.

13. Oen K, Fast M, Postl B. **Epidemiology of juvenile rheumatoid arthritis in Manitoba, Canada, 1975–92: cycles in incidence.** *J Rheumatol* 1995; 22:745–750.

14. Laxer R. *Hospital for Sick Children Atlas of Pediatrics.* Edited by R Laxer, EL Ford-Jones, J Friedman *et al.* Philadelphia, PA: Current Medicine, Inc; 2005.

15. Symmons DP, Jones M, Osborne J *et al.* **Pediatric rheumatology in the United Kingdom: data from the British Pediatric Rheumatology Group National Diagnostic Register.** *J Rheumatol* 1996; 23:1975–1980.

16. Malleson PN, Fung MY, Rosenberg AM. **The incidence of pediatric rheumatic diseases: results from the Canadian Pediatric Rheumatology Association Disease Registry.** *J Rheumatol* 1996; 23:1981–1987.

17. Gare BA, Fasth A. **The natural history of juvenile chronic arthritis: a population based cohort study. I. Onset and disease process.** *J Rheumatol* 1995; 22:295–307.

18. Bowyer S, Roettcher P. **Pediatric rheumatology clinic populations in the United States: results from a 3 year survey. Pediatric Rheumatology Database Research Group.** *J Rheumatol* 1996; 23:1968–1974.

19. Lambert JR AB, Stephenson E. **Psoriatic arthritis in childhood.** *Clin Rheum Dis* 1976; 2:339–352.

20. Calabro JJ. **Psoriatic arthritis in children.** *Arthritis Rheum* 1977; 20:415–416.

21. Sills EM. **Psoriatic arthritis in childhood.** *Johns Hopkins Med J* 1980; 146:49–53.

22. Wesolowska H. **Clinical course of psoriatic arthropathy in children.** *Mater Med Pol* 1985; 17:185–187.

23. *Textbook of Pediatric Rheumatology (Fifth Edition).* Edited by JT Cassidy, RE Petty, RM Laxer *et al.* Elsevier Saunders, 2005.

24. Huemer C, Malleson PN, Cabral DA *et al.* **Patterns of joint involvement at onset differentiate oligoarticular juvenile psoriatic arthritis from pauciarticular juvenile rheumatoid arthritis.** *J Rheumatol* 2002; 29:1531–1535.

25. McGonagle D. **Imaging the joint and enthesis: insights into pathogenesis of psoriatic arthritis.** *Ann Rheum Dis* 2005; 64(Suppl 2):ii58–ii60.

26. Hull RG. **Management guidelines for arthritis in children.** *Rheumatology* 2001; 40:1308.

27. Kane D, Balint PV, Sturrock R *et al.* **Musculoskeletal ultrasound – a state of the art review in rheumatology. Part 1: Current controversies and issues in the development of musculoskeletal ultrasound in rheumatology.** *Rheumatology* 2004; 43:823–828.

28. Doria AS, Kiss MH, Lotito AP *et al.* **Juvenile rheumatoid arthritis of the knee: evaluation with contrast-enhanced color Doppler ultrasound.** *Pediatr Radiol* 2001; 31:524–531.

29. El-Miedany YM, Housny IH, Mansour HM *et al.* **Ultrasound versus MRI in the evaluation of juvenile idiopathic arthritis of the knee.** *Joint Bone Spine* 2001; 68:222–230.

30. Giannini EH, Brewer EJ, Kuzmina N *et al.* **Methotrexate in resistant juvenile rheumatoid arthritis. Results of the U.S.A.–U.S.S.R. double-blind, placebo-controlled trial. The Pediatric Rheumatology Collaborative Study Group and The Cooperative Children's Study Group.** *N Engl J Med* 1992; 326:1043–1049.

31. Wallace CA. **The use of methotrexate in childhood rheumatic diseases.** *Arthritis Rheum* 1998; **41**:381–391.

32. Giannini EH, Cassidy JT, Brewer EJ *et al.* **Comparative efficacy and safety of advanced drug therapy in children with juvenile rheumatoid arthritis.** *Semin Arthritis Rheum* 1993; **23**:34–46.

33. Allen RC, Gross KR, Laxer RM *et al.* **Intraarticular triamcinolone hexacetonide in the management of chronic arthritis in children.** *Arthritis Rheum* 1986; **29**:997–1001.

34. Zulian F, Martini G, Gobber D *et al.* **Triamcinolone acetonide and hexacetonide intra-articular treatment of symmetrical joints in juvenile idiopathic arthritis: a double-blind trial.** *Rheumatology* 2004; **43**:1288–1291.

35. Sherry DD, Stein LD, Reed AM *et al.* **Prevention of leg length discrepancy in young children with pau-** ciarticular juvenile rheumatoid arthritis by treatment with intraarticular steroids. *Arthritis Rheum* 1999; **42**:2330–2334.

36. NICE Guidance. **Etanercept for the treatment of juvenile idiopathic arthritis.** 2002:(no 35). Available at: *www.nice.org.uk/page.aspx?o=ta035#documents.*

37. Lovell DJ, Giannini EH, Reiff A *et al.* **Etanercept in children with polyarticular juvenile rheumatoid arthritis. Pediatric Rheumatology Collaborative Study Group.** *N Engl J Med* 2000; **342**:763–769.

38. Lovell DJ, Giannini EH, Reiff A *et al.* **Long-term efficacy and safety of etanercept in children with polyarticular-course juvenile rheumatoid arthritis: interim results from an ongoing multicenter, open-label, extended-treatment trial.** *Arthritis Rheum* 2003; **48**:218–226.

7
The Management of Psoriatic Arthritis

Philip J. Mease

The management of psoriatic arthritis (PsA) begins with education. Each consultation provides an opportunity for the physician to counsel the patient and family about the disease and its clinical course that is unique to that individual. It is a chance for the patient and family to learn and adapt. There are also a variety of further ways for instruction to occur. In addition to regional educational symposia, there exists an international network of service organizations, focused on education and advocacy for patients with psoriasis and PsA, which are accessible by phone, mail, and the internet. Examples include the National Psoriasis Foundation and Arthritis Foundation in the USA, and a variety of similar organizations in other parts of the world.

There are numerous non-medication therapeutic approaches. Helping a patient cope with pain, physical dysfunction, and the embarrassment of skin lesions is achieved through counseling and understanding. It is helpful to encourage a balance of work, family, leisure, exercise, and rest. Proper sleep quality is important. Exercise that maintains muscle tone and flexibility, without stressing joints, can be taught. Physical and occupational therapists can manage specific physical therapies and provide assistive devices such as splints, orthotics, and walking aids. Interdisciplinary communication between healthcare providers is important.

Numerous medication approaches can be helpful to achieve the goals of reduction of pain and stiffness, improvement of function, energy, and quality of life, inhibition of disease progression in the joints, and amelioration or clearing of skin lesions. Treatment of skin diseases is discussed in Chapter 8, *Treatment of Psoriasis*. Most patients who develop PsA have already been working with a dermatologist and primary care provider for the treatment of the skin lesions of psoriasis, which usually precedes the development of PsA. This may have consisted of topical treatments or ultraviolet light. If the patient has been on systemic medications, such as methotrexate or a biologic, it is possible that this will have modified the initial appearance or severity of PsA. When pain in joints (arthritis) or at tendon or ligament insertion sites (enthesitis) begins, it is very common for the patient to try an over-the-counter remedy such as acetaminophen or a nonsteroidal anti-inflammatory drug (NSAID). In some cases, if there are few joints involved and the disease is mild, this may prove to be adequate. On occasion, if one or two joints are inflamed out of proportion to others, intra-articular injection with a corticosteroid may be helpful to quiet the joint down. In patients with moderate-to-severe disease, including those who do not respond adequately to NSAID or injection therapy, it will be appropriate to use a disease-modifying antirheumatic drug (DMARD). Examples include the older drugs, which non-specifically diminish immunologic over-reactivity, such as methotrexate, sulfasalazine, and cyclosporine. Whereas a pattern of drug rotation has been a common approach in psoriasis treatment in order to avoid 'wearing off' of effect and avoiding toxicity, this is not an appropriate paradigm in arthritis management, where progressive joint destruction can occur without continuous therapy. There has been scant controlled trial evidence for the efficacy of these medications in PsA (although there is substantial evidence in rheumatoid arthritis [RA]), but, nonetheless, they have been used widely, particularly methotrexate. The drawback of these medications in some patients is that they may not be fully successful, their efficacy may diminish over time, and, in some individuals, they may yield unacceptable side effects, such as the potential for hepatotoxicity with methotrexate.

An increased understanding of the specific cellular pathophysiology of the inflammatory immunologic conditions, such as RA and psoriasis, has led to the development of targeted treatments known as biologics. These are proteins biologically engineered to interact with specific cellular receptors or messengers to inhibit or downregulate overly reactive immune functions. When employed in chronic inflammatory conditions, they have proved highly efficacious in the majority of patients in both the joints and skin. Side effects do occur, such as the potential for increased infection, but with appropriate surveillance, they have so far proven to be relatively safe. Furthermore, for the first time in PsA, there is evidence that at least one class of these medications, the anti-tumor necrosis factor agents, can inhibit the progression of PsA as measured by X-ray changes over time. It is likely that this will be shown with other classes of biologics as well. This is a key goal for patients with more severe and advancing disease.

Coupled with the development of new therapeutic options has come an increased interest in developing and utilizing outcome measures in clinical trials that can accurately measure the efficacy of these medications. This is particularly important to know as we use health resources to pay for medications and monitor for adverse effects. In addition to measuring easily quantifiable benefits, such as reduction in tender and swollen joint count as well as skin lesions, it is important to measure less easily assessed benefits, such as a decrease in fatigue, improvement of quality of life, and socioeconomic benefits to the society of improved health in an individual. The measures used in PsA trials are described in the accompanying figures. International consortia of PsA and psoriasis researchers, such as the Group for Research and Assessment of Psoriasis and Psoriatic Arthritis (GRAPPA), are actively working on these measures. Other work of this group includes the development of long-term clinical registries to track disease natural history, the impacts of therapy, and treatment side effects.

At the present time, we have a growing number of therapeutic agents that can bring us closer to our goal of decreasing debilitating pain and stiffness, improving function and quality of life, improving skin disease, and inhibiting joint destruction. We have more tools that can be used either singularly or in combination to achieve optimal benefit at various stages of disease. Measuring benefit of these therapies is an evolving science. The accompanying figures detail these options. Combining use of these agents with increased understanding of the disease and increased public awareness through education provides great promise for the treatment of patients with PsA and psoriasis.

Therapy of PsA

- Education
- Physical therapy and exercise
- Splints and assistive devices
- NSAIDs
- DMARDs
- Biologic agents
- Intra-articular corticosteroid injections
- Surgery: joint revision or replacement

FIGURE 7.1. Patient education is an important component of management of psoriatic arthritis (PsA). Not only may the patient and family obtain information from their physicians and nurses, but also by phone, mail, or online from patient service organizations devoted to psoriasis or arthritis. These organizations are devoted to education, support and advocacy for patients with PsA and psoriasis. In the USA, the National Psoriasis Foundation (*www. psoriasis.org*) and the Arthritis Foundation (*www.arthritis.org*) are two of these. Joint preservation techniques can help avoid overuse of painful joints. Modification of daily activities and of the workplace environment may do the same. Occupational therapists can direct patients toward adaptive equipment, such as large-handled cutlery. Physical therapy, such as hydrotherapy, may be beneficial, and isometric exercises can help maintain joint strength and flexibility. Non-steriodal antiinflammatory drugs (NSAIDs [eg, ibuprofen, diclofenac, and naproxen]) and the newer cyclooxygenase (COX)-2 NSAIDs (eg, celecoxib) have traditionally been the drugs first used. Many patients respond well to NSAIDs alone. Caution must be exercised regarding gastrointestinal side effects, which can be problematic, or cardiovascular risk in susceptible patients, which may limit their acceptability to patients. In addition, some patients rarely experience worsening of psoriasis with NSAIDs. Disease-modifying antirheumatic drugs (DMARDs), such as methotrexate and sulfasalazine, are often used in conjunction with NSAIDs for severe articular disease, but side effects can affect patient tolerability. Although these drugs may control the acute inflammation of PsA they do not significantly affect progression of radiologic or clinical damage. New, more effective drugs have been sought for some time and some of the problems inherent in the treatment of PsA may be addressed by the new biologic agents, including those that target tumor necrosis factor (TNF), which plays a central role in the inflammatory process in PsA. Intra-articular corticosteroid injections may be useful when one or two joints are flaring. If a joint has been sufficiently damaged, it may be necessary to enlist an orthopedic surgeon to perform revisional or replacement surgery.

Therapeutic targets in PsA

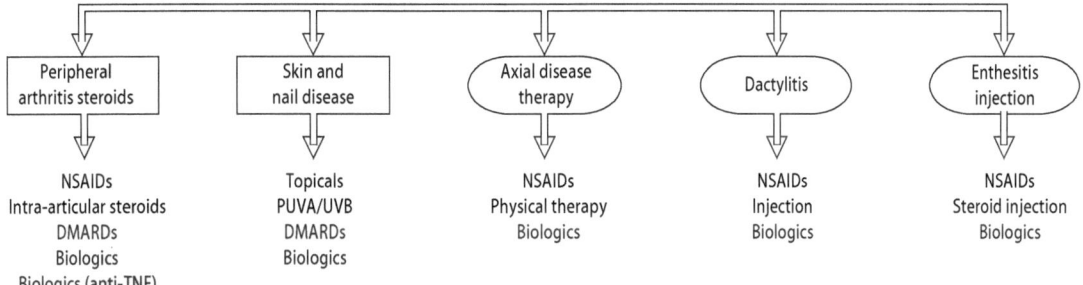

FIGURE 7.2. There are a number of different 'targets' to consider when choosing treatments for PsA. These include the peripheral (non-spine) joints, the skin and nails, the spine, dactylitis ('sausage digits'), and enthesitis (insertion sites of tendons, ligaments, and joint capsule). When more than one of these targets are inflamed and/or damaged in PsA, one needs to think about the optimal approach to managing each area, as well as thinking about the patient as a whole. Listed under each target are examples of therapies that may possibly be helpful. There is not enough evidence from clinical trials to inform us whether certain therapies will be effective; for example, DMARDs in the context of axial (spine) disease, dactylitis, or enthesis. There is evidence from studies in ankylosing spondylitis, a related spondyloarthropathy, that DMARDs can be effective in peripheral joints but not the spine, so until there are specific data for PsA in this regard, we tend to extrapolate from our evidence in related conditions. PUVA, combination of psoralen (P) and long-wave ultraviolet radiation (UVA); UVB, middle-wave ultraviolet radiation. Reproduced with kind permission of Artie Kavanaugh, University of California, San Diego.

Who will progress aggressively?

- Presenting elements to consider:
  - lack of response to NSAIDs
  - number of joints involved
  - erosions on radiograph
  - elevated sedimentation rate or CRP
  - disability

- Observation over time:
  - inadequate response to serial therapy trials
  - progression of erosions on radiograph

FIGURE 7.3. Treatment decisions require consideration of disease that may progress aggressively. Predictors of aggressive disease include a poor response to NSAIDs therapy, polyarthritis, radiographic erosions, elevated sedimentation rate, and C-reactive protein (CRP), and noticeable disability resulting from PsA. Over time, aggressive progression of disease is indicated by an inadequate response to trials of serial therapy and radiographic progression of erosions. Modified with permission from [1].

Measures of PsA outcome

- ACR response criteria: 20%, 50%, 70% (validated in RA, not PsA):
  - tender and swollen joint count (modified for PsA to include DIP and CMC joints: 78/76, 68/66)
  - 3/5: patient global, physician global, patient pain, HAQ, acute phase reactant (sedimentation rate, CRP)
- PsARC:
  - improvement in at least 2 of 4 criteria, including:
    - Physician Global Assessment (0–5);
    - Patient Global Assessment (0–5);
    - tender joint score (≥30%); and
    - swollen joint score (≥30%)
  - improvement in at least 1 of 2 joint scores
  - no worsening in any criteria
- DAS
- Enthesitis score
- Dactylitis score
- Function/QoL/disability indices (HAQ, SF-36, DLQI, PsAQoL)
- Radiographic (modified Sharp, modified Steinbrocker, Wassenberg)
- Skin (PASI, target lesion, static global)

FIGURE 7.4. Outcome of PsA can be measured using various assessment instruments. The American College of Rheumatology (ACR) clinical response criteria are categorized according to percentage reductions (20%, 50%, or 70%) in tender and swollen joint counts and in three or more of patient pain assessment, patient global assessment, physician global assessment, patient disability assessment (using the Health Assessment Questionnaire [HAQ]), and acute phase reactant. The Psoriatic Arthritis Response Criteria (PsARC) was first crafted for a study of sulfasalazine [2] and named when used in the first etanercept trial [3]. Both have been used in PsA trials, proving to be discriminative and responsive. The disease activity score (DAS), developed in Europe as a measure both of the current state of rheumatoid arthritis (RA) as well as change of RA with therapy, has been shown to be a highly sensitive and specific instrument when analyzed retrospectively in etanercept and infliximab trials (Antoni C and Mease P, personal communication).

Scoring systems to measure change of enthesitis and dactylitis with therapy are in development. Function can be measured using the HAQ. Quality of life can be measured using the Short Form 36 (SF-36), Dermatology Life Quality Index (DLQI), or PsA Quality of Life (PsAQoL) questionnaire. Radiographic assessment is a developing science in PsA, with recent trials employing the modified Sharp or modified van der Heijde–Sharp systems, which have been used in RA. Skin lesions can be quantified using the Psoriasis Area and Severity Index (PASI) and the target lesion score. PASI is a composite measure of erythema, scale and induration, weighted by severity and body surface area. The target lesion score is derived from the scale, plaque, and erythema of a single lesion. The static global is a less quantitative overall assessment that uses phrases such as 'clear' or 'almost clear'. CMC, carpometacarpal; DIP, distal interphalangeal. Modified with permission from [4].

Trial-verified benefit of traditional DMARDs in PsA

Compound	Arthritis	Skin
Sulfasalazine (5*)	Marginal	None
Methotrexate (1*)	Improvement in Physician Global Assessment only	Improvement in area of skin involvement only
Cyclosporine (abs.)	Marginal	Good
	Marginal	None
Gold (1*)	Marginal	None
Azathioprine (1*)	PsARC 59%	Median PASI
Leflunomide (1*)	ACR20 36.3%	Improvement 23.8%

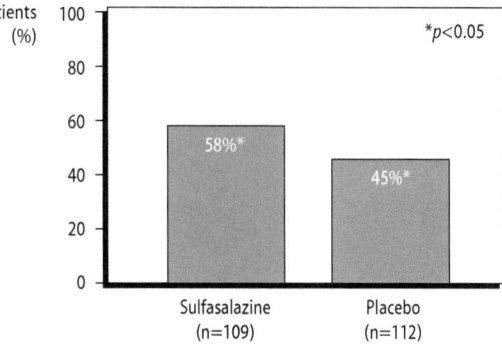

Sulfasalazine in PsA: PsARC response at 36 weeks

FIGURE 7.5. Disease-modifying drugs are those which interfere with basic biologic pathways in cells. Although they may effect a number of cell types nondiscriminately, they are given in order to have the greatest impact on rapidly proliferating inflammatory cells. The effects of DMARDs in patients with PsA have been measured in various controlled studies. Sulfasalazine was found to have a marginal affect on arthritis and no effect on the skin in PsA [2]. Methotrexate improved arthritis according to Physician Global Assessment only and improved the area of skin involvement only [5]. This study did not enroll an adequate number of patients to calculate adequate statistical significance, and only a third of the patients used a methotrexate dose currently considered adequate, so it is probably not a fair reflection of the capability of this medication in PsA. Cyclosporine had a marginal effect on arthritis and a good benefit on the skin [6]. Both gold and azathioprine had a marginal effect on arthritis and no benefit on the skin in patients with PsA [7,8]. The most recent trial, that of leflunomide, was well designed, adequately powered, and showed statistically significant superiority of leflunomide compared with placebo in both joints and skin [9]. Traditionally, these drugs are used for RA, and thus they have been extended to patients with PsA, but the results of these studies suggest that they may not be adequately effective in many PsA patients and new therapies are needed. ACR20, American College of Rheumatology 20% improvement criteria.

FIGURE 7.6. Effect of sulfasalazine on PsA was measured in a double-blind randomized placebo-controlled trial [2]. Patients with NSAID-resistant PsA were randomly allocated to receive sulfasalazine 2000 mg/day or placebo and were followed for 36 weeks. Treatment response was based on joint pain/tenderness and swelling scores and physician and patient global assessments. At the end of treatment, response rates were 58% for sulfasalazine and 45% for placebo. The primary outcome measure of PsARC was statistically significant, but treatment differences favoring sulfasalazine in the four components that defined PsARC response were each statistically weaker. Adverse reactions were fewer than expected and were primarily gastrointestinal complaints, including dyspepsia, nausea, vomiting, and diarrhea. A longitudinal analysis (including data over the treatment period) showed a weaker treatment effect than did the last visit analysis. Sulfasalazine compared with placebo percentage response at 36 months showed no significant difference ($p = 0.13$). Modified with permission from [2].

Leflunomide in PsA: ACR20 and PsARC results

a) ACR20

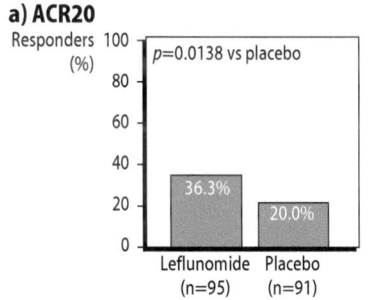

b) PsARC

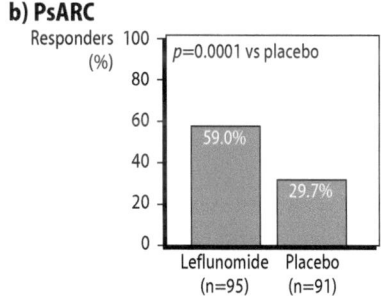

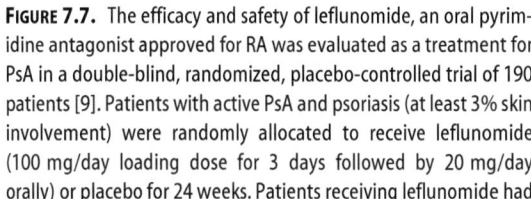

FIGURE 7.7. The efficacy and safety of leflunomide, an oral pyrimidine antagonist approved for RA was evaluated as a treatment for PsA in a double-blind, randomized, placebo-controlled trial of 190 patients [9]. Patients with active PsA and psoriasis (at least 3% skin involvement) were randomly allocated to receive leflunomide (100 mg/day loading dose for 3 days followed by 20 mg/day orally) or placebo for 24 weeks. Patients receiving leflunomide had significantly better ACR20 **(a)** and PsARC **(b)** scores than patients receiving placebo. In addition, patients receiving leflunomide showed significant improvement in the designated psoriasis target lesion and mean changes from baseline in PASI scores and quality-of-life assessments. Diarrhea and liver function test abnormalities occurred at higher rates in patients receiving leflunomide. Modified with permission from [9].

Pathophysiology of PsA

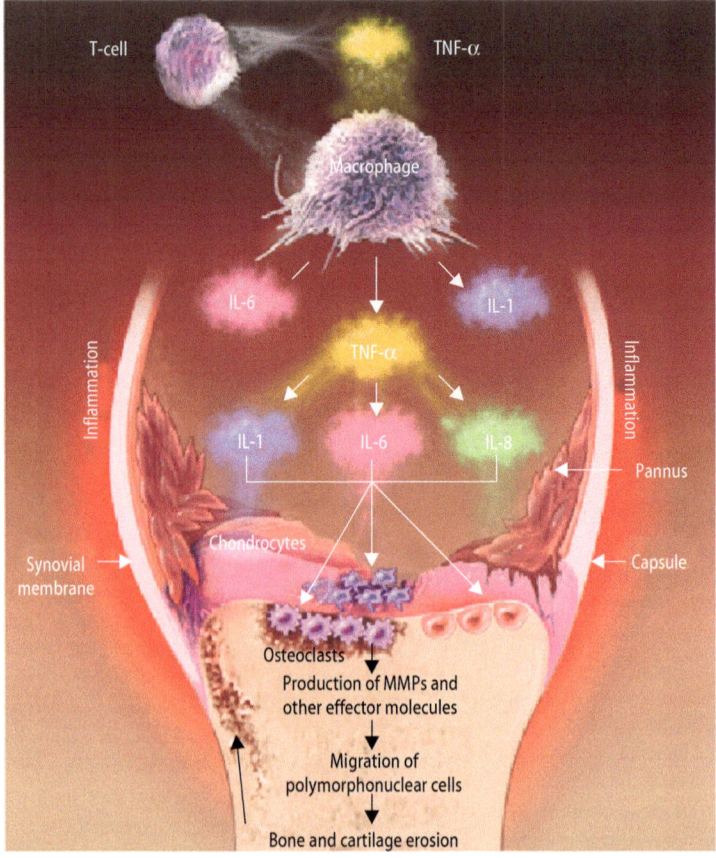

FIGURE 7.8. A number of cells and molecular messengers (cytokines and chemokines) are involved in the pathogenesis of disease in both the joints and the skin in patients with PsA. Prominently involved effector cells are T-lymphocytes and macrophages, which become activated due to antigen stimulation. A variety of pro-inflammatory cytokines are generated, including TNF-alpha (TNF-α), interleukin (IL)-1, IL-6 and IL-8, and others, which in turn, interact with fibroblasts and chondrocytes to generate enzymes responsible for cartilage destruction and contribute to the differentiation of osteoclasts, which cause bone destruction. One of the key cytokines, TNF-α, is a pro-inflammatory cytokine, which can be detected in high levels in psoriatic skin lesions and in the joints of patients with PsA. Monocytes secrete TNF-α, usually in response to injury or infection, and this cytokine displays multiple biologic activities. At the cellular level, TNF-α is involved in stimulation of collagenase and prostaglandin E_2 synthesis and production of other cytokines, including IL-1, IL-6, and IL-8. At the tissue level, TNF-α is involved in proteoglycan breakdown and bone resorption. Some or all of these processes may play a part in the pathogenesis of PsA. An increased understanding of this inflammatory cascade has opened the door to the development of specifically targeted therapies that can inhibit the cascade, resulting in greater effectiveness and potentially fewer side effects. MMP, matrix metalloproteinase.

Role of cytokines and cytokine inhibitors in chronic inhibition

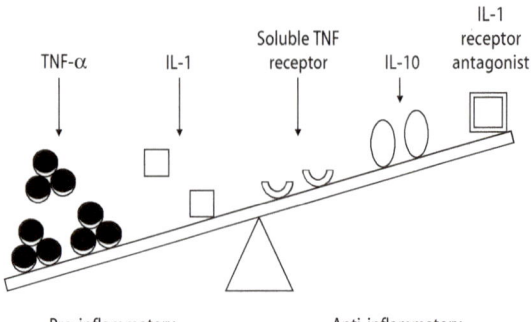

FIGURE 7.9. Pro-inflammatory cytokines, such as TNF-α and IL-1, are commonly found at high levels in the tissue of patients with chronic inflammatory diseases such as PsA [10]. This is counterbalanced to an extent by increased production of anti-inflammatory cytokines such as soluble TNF receptor, IL-10 and IL-1 receptor antagonist. However, the upregulation of homeostatic regulatory mechanisms is not sufficient and the anti-inflammatory mediators are unable to neutralize all of the TNF-α and IL-1 produced. It is thought that the pro-inflammatory cytokines are linked in a network, with TNF-α playing a significant role, making this a logical therapeutic target.

Key actions attributed to TNF

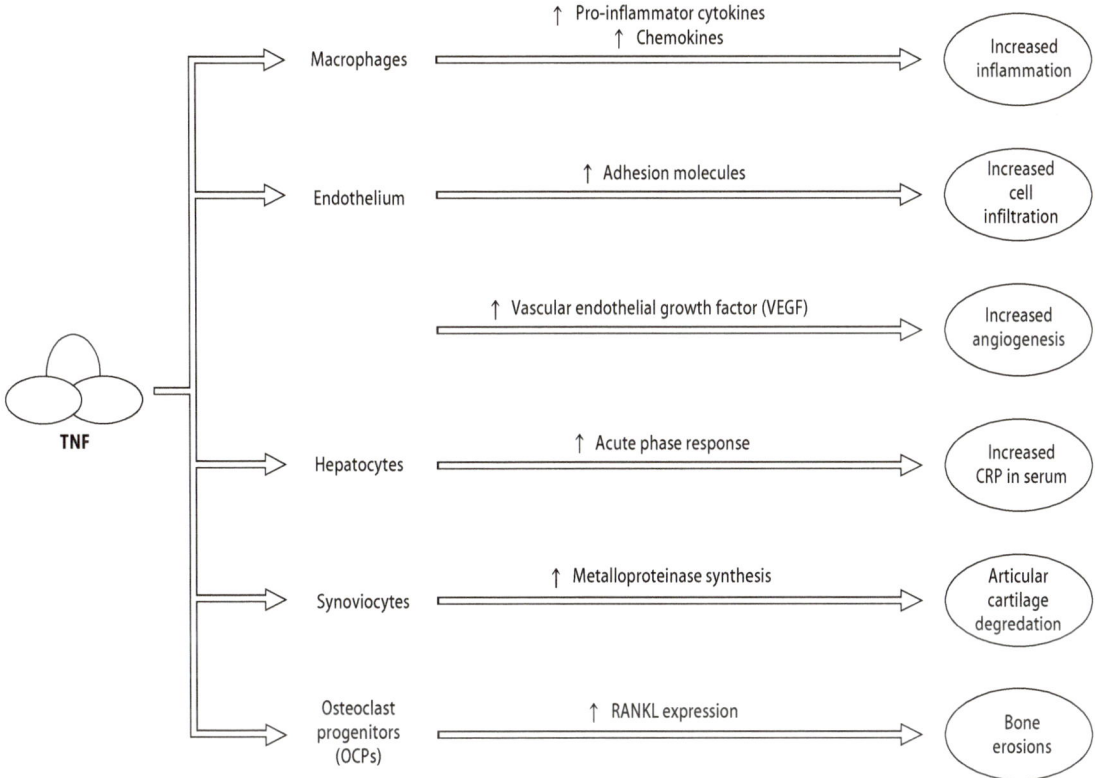

FIGURE 7.10. TNF is thought to be involved in several key actions that would potentiate the pathologic processes seen in PsA. Stimulation of pro-inflammatory cytokines and chemokines would cause increased inflammation. Increased expression of endothelial adhesion molecules would potentiate cell infiltration and greater vascular endothelial growth factor secretion would lead to increased angiogenesis. A heightened acute phase response would cause the elevated CRP levels that are commonly found in PsA. Increased metalloproteinase synthesis would cause articular cartilage degradation, and increased expression of the receptor activator of NF-κB ligand (RANKL) would lead to bone erosions.

Cytokine inhibition

a)

Soluble receptor

Monoclonal antibody

No signal

b)

Receptor antagonist

Monoclonal antibody

No signal

FIGURE 7.11. **(a)** One possible method of cytokine inhibition is to neutralize the cytokine, such as TNF, by binding it to a monoclonal antibody. This would then prevent the cytokine from binding with its soluble receptor, which in turn would send no signal to the target cell. **(b)** Alternatively, cytokines may be inhibited by blocking their cell-bound receptors, either with a receptor antagonist or with a monoclonal antibody. Both can bind to cell-bound receptors, which in turn would send no signal to the target cell. Modified with permission from [11].

TNF inihibition

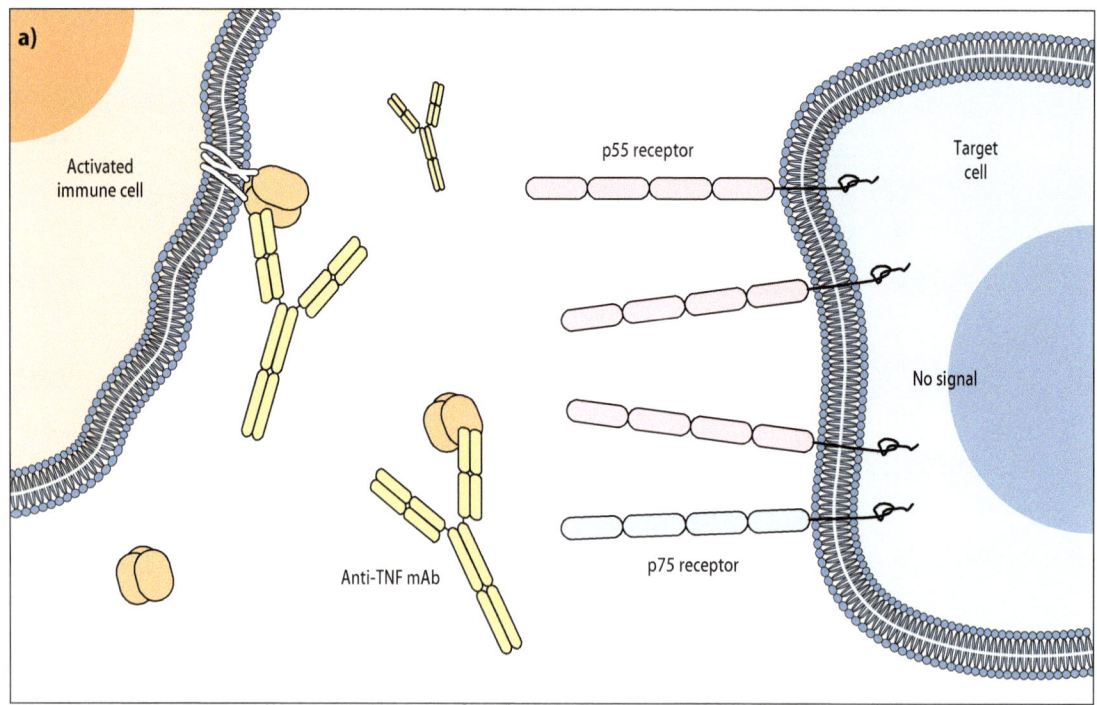

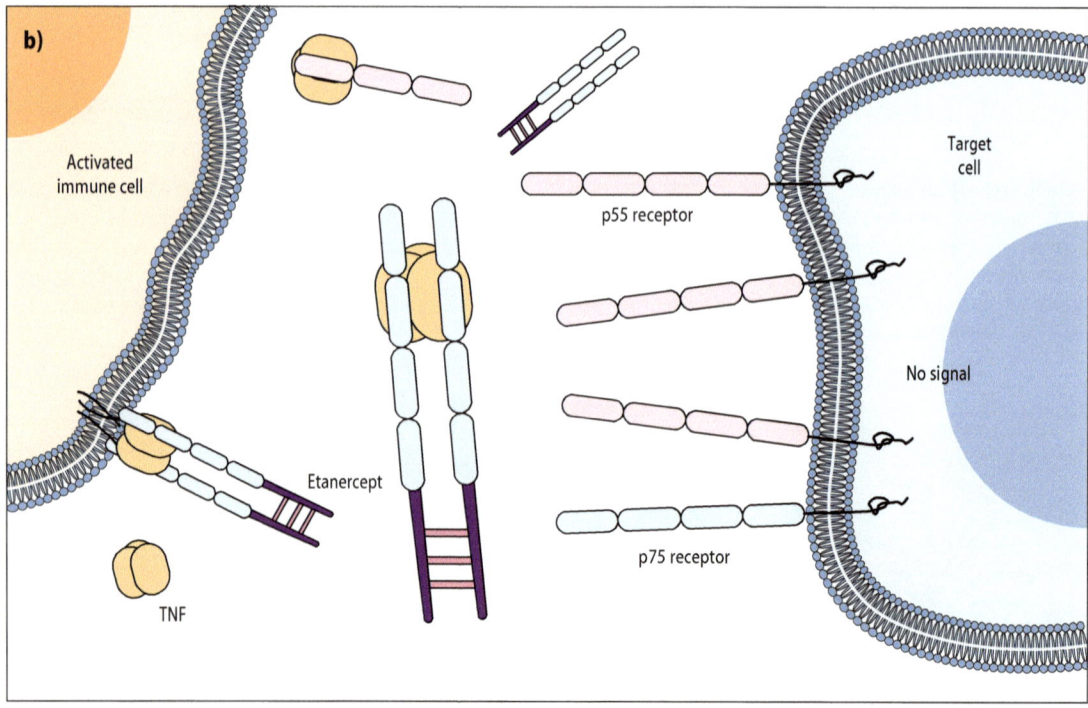

FIGURE 7.12. TNF inhibition. TNF binds to cell-bound TNF receptors. There are two distinct but structurally similar receptors, designated p55 and p75. The receptors form dimers on the cell surface, where each binds one molecule of TNF, thus initiating a signal. Soluble forms of both the p55 and p75 receptor have been identified. **(a)** Anti-TNF monoclonal antibodies (mAbs) can bind to cell-bound and soluble TNF, preventing binding with the p55 and p75 receptors on target cells, which in turn are not activated. Examples of such mAbs include the chimeric agent, infliximab, and the fully human adalimumab. **(b)** Alternatively, TNF may be inhibited using soluble receptors. Etanercept is a recombinant dimeric form of the soluble TNF p75 receptor. Like the endogenous soluble receptor, etanercept binds tightly to TNF, rendering it inactive and preventing any signal in the target cell.

Design elements in current PsA trials

- ≥3 tender and swollen joints (in all but infliximab trials):
  - allows evaluation of patients with oligoarticular presentation <5 tender and swollen joints
- Variable amount of skin involvement
- Background methotrexate allowed, not required, and typically used in 40–50% of patients
- Low-dose prednisone allowed, but rarely used
- Key measures: ACR, PsARC, PASI response
- Assessment domains in development:
  - spine
  - enthesitis
  - dactylitis
  - fatigue
  - function/QoL
  - radiologic progression

FIGURE 7.13. Prior to the current interest in treating PsA with biologic agents, there were few controlled trials, and little standardization of study design or outcome measures. However, with recent increased interest in treatment of PsA, because of the promise of effectiveness of newer medicines, more standardized study approaches have been employed. In most trials, patients with at least three tender and swollen joints are included, a lower minimum number than allowed in RA trials, so that the experience of patients with oligoarticular joint involvement can be determined. Since joint response is the primary outcome in these trials, some patients may be entered who have less than 10% body surface area involvement with psoriasis, the usual minimum for a pure psoriasis trial. Since assessment instruments used for the skin do not perform as reliably in patients with minimal skin involvement, evaluations are focused on patients with higher amounts of skin disease who are evaluable for PASI scoring (≥3% body surface area involvement). For ethical reasons, for those having partial response to methotrexate, continuation of this is allowed and the patients are then stratified, based on methotrexate use, to new treatment or placebo. In most studies, background methotrexate is used in 40–50% of patients. Background NSAIDs use is allowed, as is low-dose prednisone, although the latter is rarely used because of concern regarding potential flare of psoriasis after steroids are discontinued. The key measures of response have been the ACR, PsARC, and PASI responses. Variably, other measures in development have been performed, as noted.

FIGURE 7.14. Following an encouraging phase II study of etanercept in PsA, showing highly significant ACR, PsARC, and PASI responses [3], a larger multi-center study was conducted.

Demographics of the patient population in this phase III trial are shown in this figure [12]. These demographics have proven to be similar in other trials discussed in this chapter. A total of 205 patients with PsA and psoriasis were enrolled in the study; 101 received etanercept and 104 received placebo. As mentioned previously, randomization was stratified by concomitant methotrexate use. Patients received 25 mg etanercept or placebo for 24 weeks [12]. Arthritis severity was measured by ACR20 and the PsARC. Psoriasis activity was measured by improvement in target lesion score in all patients and, in a subset of patients with ≥3% body surface area involvement with psoriasis lesions (n = 62 for placebo; n = 66 for etanercept), by using the PASI. Modified with permission from [12].

Demographics of etanercept phase III trial

Characteristic	Placebo (n=104)	Etanercept (n=101)
Age (range)	47 (21–73)	48 (18–76)
Sex (male/female, %)	45/55	57/43
Arthritis duration (mean years)	9.2	9.0
Psoriasis duration (mean years)	19.7	18.3
Concomitant medications:		
Corticosteroids	15%	19%
NSAIDs	83%	88%
Methotrexate	41%	42%
Mean weekly dose	15.4 mg	16.3 mg

Results of phase III trial of etanercept in PsA

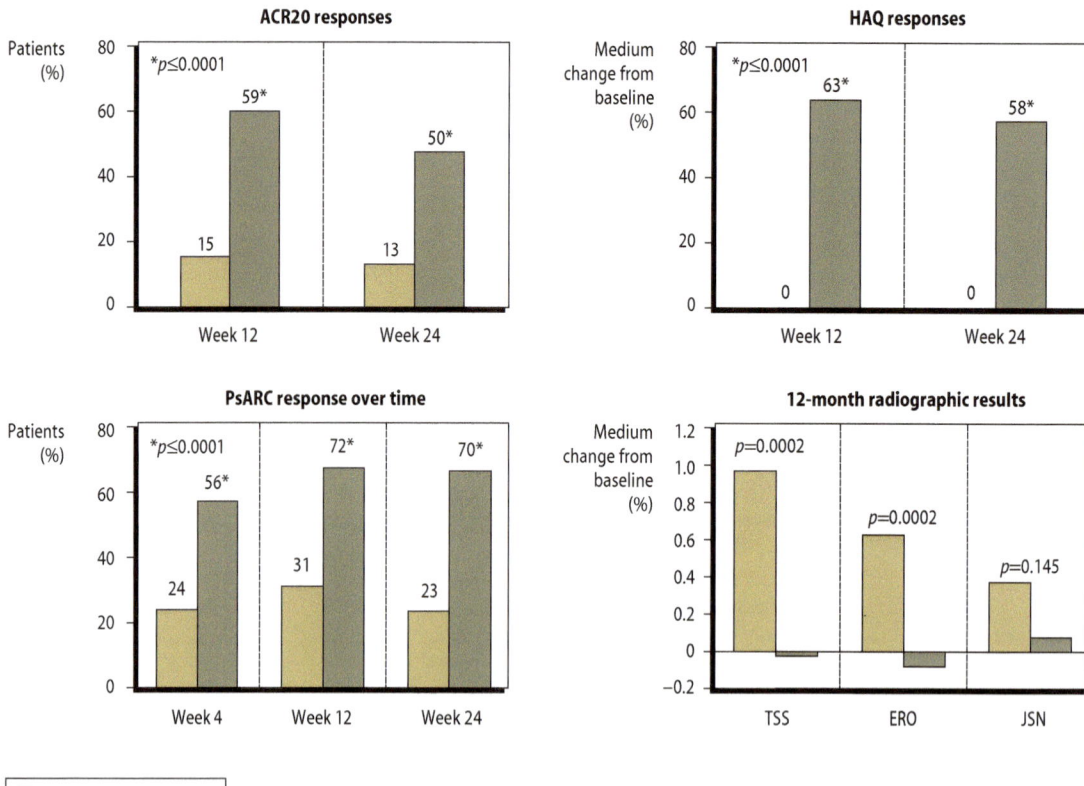

FIGURE 7.15. The primary endpoint, ACR20 response at 12 weeks, was met by 59% of patients receiving etanercept and 15% of patients receiving placebo (p < 0.001) [12]. Patients receiving etanercept had significantly greater responses in each of the parameters of disease activity compared with placebo, regardless of concomitant methotrexate use. ACR20 response is considered by many investigators to be a more demanding arthritis efficacy endpoint than the PsARC because of the large number of elements that must be improved to achieve an ACR response. The clinical response for etanercept was maintained through 6 months and 70% of patients enrolled in the open-label extension trial achieved ACR20 by 12 months, suggesting that etanercept provided durable relief of symptoms. Patients treated with etanercept showed significantly more improvement in target lesions than patients treated with placebo; the median improvement in target lesion at 24 weeks was 33% in patients receiving etanercept compared with 0% in patients receiving placebo. Results from the subset of patients who were evaluated using PASI showed a median improvement of 47% in patients receiving etanercept while no improvement was seen in those receiving placebo. Patients treated with etanercept had significant improvement in HAQ and SF-36 scores [12]. Etanercept was well tolerated, with no increase in the number of serious adverse events occurring in patients receiving etanercept compared with those receiving placebo. At 12 months, it was demonstrated that patients treated with etanercept showed no radiographic progression, as illustrated by total Sharp score (TSS), erosion score (ERO), or joint space narrowing (JSN) score. In contrast, patients who received placebo showed significant progression in these parameters [12]. Modified with permission from [12].

FIGURE 7.16. Durability of anti-TNF effect on inhibition of joint destruction observed at 2 years. In the open-label extension phase of the etanercept phase III study in PsA, it was demonstrated that there continued to be an inhibition of progressive joint destruction as measured by lack of radiographic change. This was seen in both the originally etanercept-treated group as well as the originally placebo-treated group once they were on etanercept therapy. *$p = 0.0006$, stratified rank test; [†]$p = 0.0006$, stratified rank test.

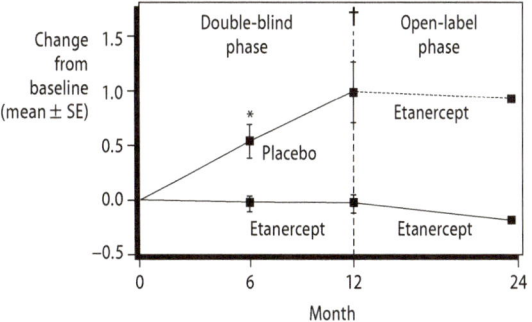

Etanercept in PsA: radiographic progression mean change in TSS through 24 months

FIGURE 7.17. Study design of the phase III Infliximab Multinational Psoriatic Arthritis Controlled Trial 2 (IMPACT 2) involving 200 patients randomized to infliximab 5 mg/kg versus placebo, stratified according to background methotrexate use (used by 46% of patients). Patients were dosed at weeks 0, 2 and 6 and every 8 weeks thereafter. Based on clinical presentation at week 16, patients could 'early escape' and if on placebo, were administered infliximab, and if on infliximab, were administered placebo. After week 24, all patients received infliximab. Demographics were similar to those of the etanercept trial [13]. Modified with permission from [13].

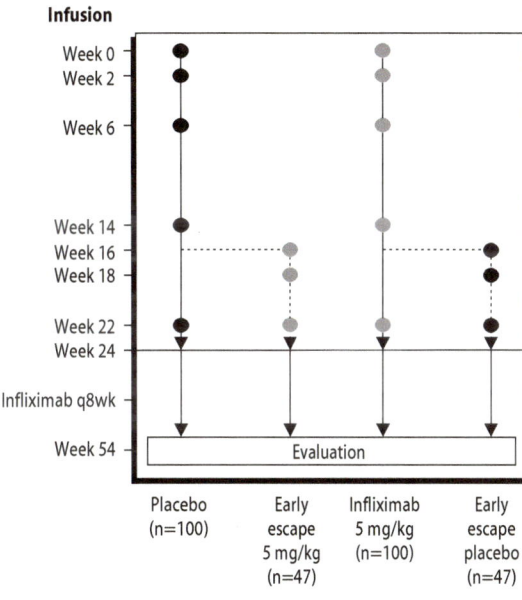

IMPACT 2: study design/subject disposition

FIGURE 7.18. The primary endpoint in the phase III infliximab study was ACR20. Additional endpoints were PsARC and PASI 75. At week 14, patients who had received treatment with infliximab showed a significantly greater response on all criteria, compared with patients who had received placebo [13]. Modified with permission from [13].

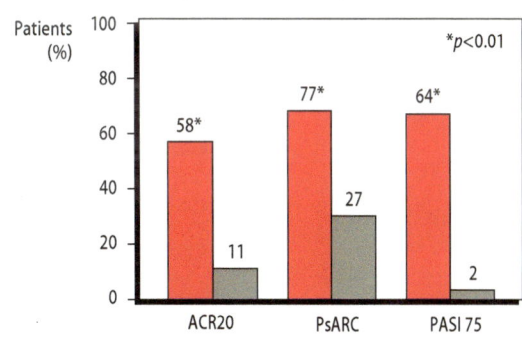

Infliximab in psoriasis/PsA therapy: phase III study

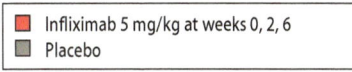

Infliximab reduces inflammation in PsA (IMPACT 2)

a) Patients with ≥1 dactylitis digits

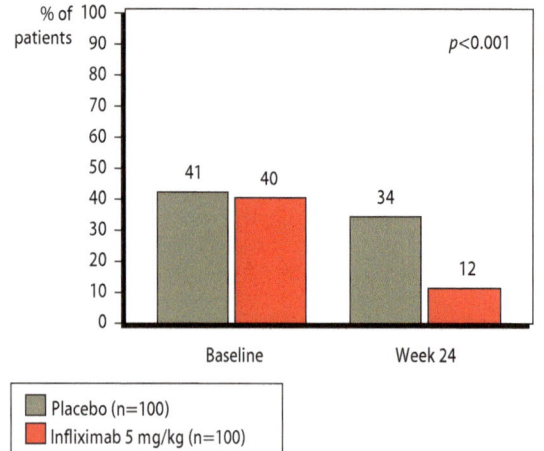

b) Patients with enthesopathy

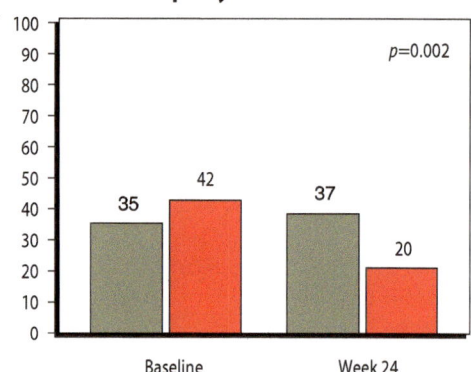

Figure 7.19. In the phase II IMPACT 2 study, the percentage of patients with ≥1 dactylitic digit was determined at baseline. (a) The percentage of patients with dactylitis diminished significantly with infliximab treatment over the course of the study.

(b) Similarly, the percentage of patients with enthesitis, as determined by palpation of tendon insertions at the heel, diminished significantly with infliximab treatment. Modified with permission from [13].

ADEPT study design

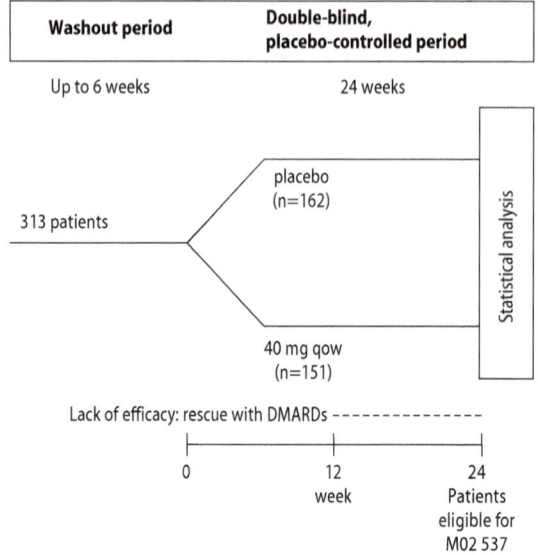

Figure 7.20. The phase III ADalimumab Effectiveness in Psoriatic arthritis Trial (ADEPT) involved 313 patients randomized to adalimumab, 40 mg every other week subcutaneously, or placebo, stratified by methotrexate background (50%). Demographics were similar to those of etanercept and infliximab studies. If an inadequate effect at week 12 was noted, adjustment of background medications could occur. The open-label phase began at week 24 [4]. Data taken from [14,15].

FIGURE 7.21. ACR responses in adalimumab phase III trial. ACR20, −50, and −70 responses were achieved in 58%, 36%, and 20% of participants at week 12, respectively, and were sustained at week 24. Data taken from [14,15].

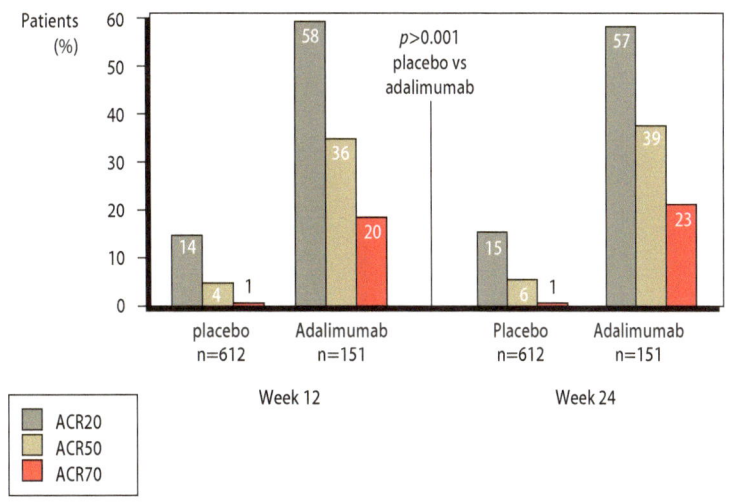

FIGURE 7.22. HAQ scores in the adalimumab phase III trial. In the adalimumab group, significant improvements were seen in the functional measure, HAQ, of 0.4 points change. The minimally important clinical difference of HAQ has been determined to be 0.3 [16]. Data taken from [14,15].

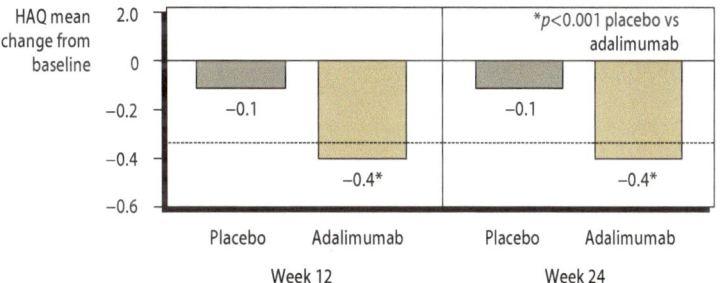

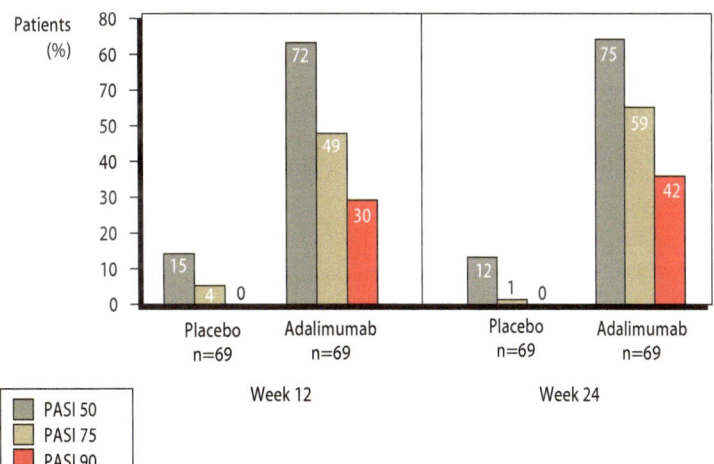

FIGURE 7.23. Highly significant improvements in psoriasis skin lesions were noted at week 12, with further improvement noted at week 24. Data taken from [14,15].

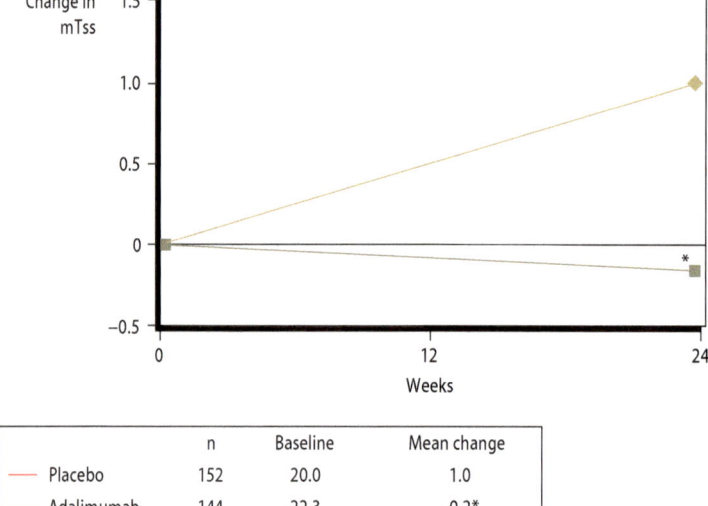

FIGURE 7.24. Of the total 313 patients with moderate to severely active PsA who participated in ADEPT, 296 patients had X-rays at baseline and week 24, and 265 patients also had X-rays at week 48 (in the open-label extension study). During the 24-week blinded study period, patients receiving adalimumab had significantly less progression in modified total Sharp score (mTSS) when compared with placebo patients (*p < 0.001, ranked analysis of covariance [ANCOVA]). Statistical significance was maintained in all sensitivity analyses. At week 24, the change in erosion scores and joint space narrowing scores were 0.6 and 0.4 for placebo patients and 0.0 and −0.2 for adalimumab-treated patients, respectively (p < 0.001, ranked ANCOVA). Neither treatment arm demonstrated significant progression in PsA-associated features, and X-rays taken at week 48 demonstrated that the lack of progression observed at week 24 was maintained to week 48 in adalimumab-treated patients. Modified with permission from [15,17].

Safety issues of anti-TNF therapy

- Laboratory assessment:
  - routine lab monitoring (eg, CBC, LFTs, creatinine); not essential unless clinically indicated
- Injection site reactions to subcutaneous medications are mild, self-limited, and do not necessitate cessation of therapy
- Infusion reactions to IV medications are rare – may necessitate slowing IV or ceasing infusion and possibly medical interventions
- Rare events:
  - severe bacterial infections
  - tuberculosis
  - other opportunistic infections (eg, histoplasmosis, coccidioidomycosis, listeria)
  - demyelinating disorders (eg, multiple sclerosis)
  - drug-induced lupus
  - congestive heart failure
  - cytopenias
- Cancer rates are not increased compared with background prevalence

---

FIGURE 7.25. Anti-TNF therapy is associated with fewer risks and serious adverse events than the more traditional DMARDs. Injection site reactions to subcutaneous medications are mild and self-limiting. Infusion reactions to intravenous (IV) medications are rare, but when they do occur, they may necessitate slowing the administration of the drug or ceasing it completely. Serious bacterial and opportunistic infections may occur. An increased incidence of tuberculosis has been seen, but its risk can be mitigated through appropriate screening. No increase in cancer rates compared with background prevalence in RA populations has been reported in patients receiving anti-TNF therapy in clinical trials in RA. There is little known about background prevalence of cancers in PsA. CBC, complete blood count; LFT, liver function test.

PsA: new therapies on the horizon

- Other anti-TNF agents (eg, CDP870)
- IL-1 Inhibitors (eg, anakinra (Kineret®), IL-1 TRAP)
- Other cytokine targets (eg, IL-6, IL-12, IL-15)
- Co-stimulatory blockade: alefacept (Amevive™; LFA-3–CD2), abatacept (CTLA-4–Ig; B7–CD28)
- B-cell ablation or modulation: rituximab (Rituxan®)
- Small molecules (eg, MAP kinase,TACE, Syk inhibitors)
- Combination therapies:
  – with DMARDs
  – with other biologics

FIGURE 7.26. The success of currently available anti-TNF medications has prompted the search for other biologic therapies for treatment of PsA. Other anti-TNF therapies include CDP870. Inhibition of other pro-inflammatory cytokines such as IL-1, IL-6, IL-12 and IL-15, currently in development, are likely to be beneficial in PsA. Agents that block costimulatory signals may be of benefit in PsA (*see* Figures 6.27 and 6.28). Ablation or modulation of B-lymphocytes is a promising approach to therapy of RA but has yet to be tested in PsA or psoriasis. A number of small molecules, taken orally, which specifically target elements in the inflammatory cascade are in development in RA and may be useful in PsA. These include mitogen-activated protein (MAP) kinase, Syk kinase and TNF-α-converting enzyme (TACE) inhibitors. All of these therapies might be used alone or in combination with DMARDs, or with other biologic agents. CTLA, cytotoxic T-lymphocyte antigen; Ig, immunoglobulin; LFA, leukocyte function-associated antigen.

T-cell activation requires two signals

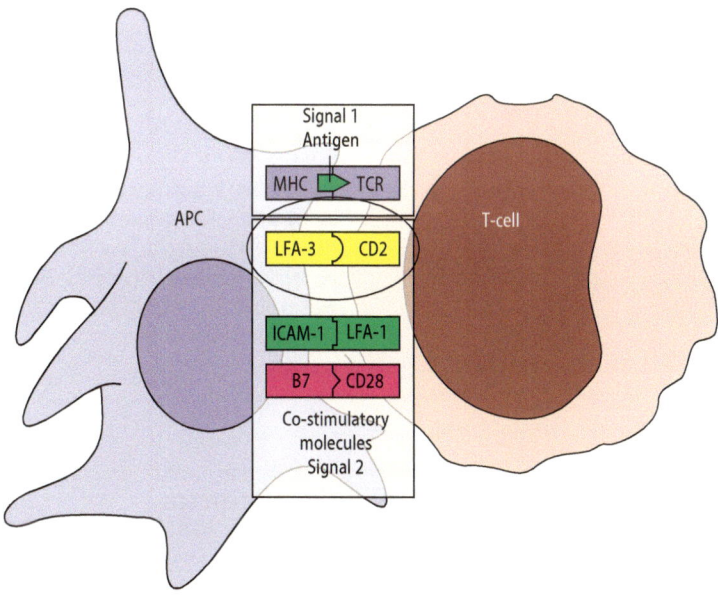

FIGURE 7.27. For a T-cell to become activated, two different signals are required to be delivered during contact with the antigen-presenting cell (APC). The first signal (signal 1) occurs on presentation of antigen by the APC to the naïve T-cell. The antigen, in association with major histocompatibility complex molecules expressed by the APC, is recognized by the T-cell receptor (TCR-CD3) on the surface of T-cells and binding occurs. Binding or pairing between cell surface molecules on naïve T-cells and APCs provides the costimulatory signal (signal 2). A protein molecule on the surface of the APC binds to a protein molecule on the surface of the T-cell. Receptor pairs important in the generation of signal 2 are leukocyte function-associated antigen (LFA)-3 with CD2, CD80 with CD28, and intracellular adhesion molecule 1 (ICAM-1) with LFA-1. Drugs have been developed to interfere with each of these pathways, including alefacept, abatacept, and efalizumab, respectively. Signal 2 can be disrupted by interference with receptor pair binding, blocking activation of T-cells, which may become anergic. Alefacept has been approved in psoriasis and has shown benefit in an open trial in PsA (*see* Figure 7.28) and results of a controlled trial, pending presentation, are positive (Mease P, personal communication). Efalizumab, also approved for psoriasis, was tested in a controlled trial in PsA and the ACR20 response was not statistically superior in the treated group, although it did show a positive trend. Abatacept, soon to be approved in RA, has yet to be tested in PsA. Modified with permission from [18].

PsA open-label study: alefacept

- LFA–IgG1 fusion protein – blocks LFA-3–CD2 interactions, thus inhibits T-cell response. Specific ablative effect on $CD45RO^+$ cells
- Proven efficacy in psoriasis
- 11 PsA patients, open label, 12.5 mg IV every week x 12 weeks
- 7/11 (64%) – ACR20; 3 (27%) – ACR50
- 7/11 (64%) – PASI 50 response
- Synovial biopsies: reduction of CD4 and CD8 cells and CD68 macrophages in synovial lining
- Transient drops of CD4 counts – monitoring required

FIGURE 7.28. Alefacept, a co-stimulatory blockade agent that blocks LFA-3-CD2 interaction (*see* Chapter 8), was assessed in 185 patients with PsA. All patients were required to be on background methotrexate. Patients were randomized 2 : 1 to receive 15 mg alefacept intramuscularly per week versus placebo for 12 weeks, at which point alefacept was discontinued and methotrexate continued. The primary endpoint of joint assessment was at 24 weeks. At this point, 54% of the alefacept-treated patients achieved an ACR20 response whereas 23% of patients not receiving alefacept did so ($p < 0.001$) [19].

Example of an adaptive aid: a wrist splint

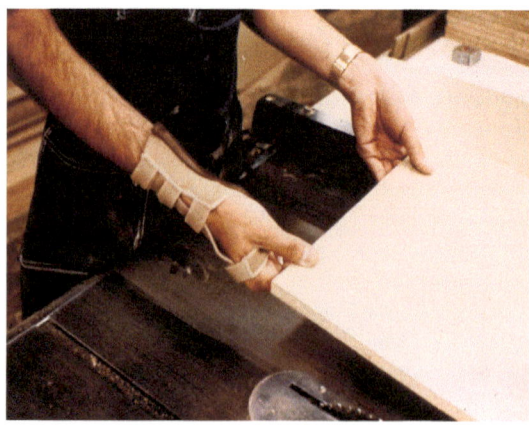

FIGURE 7.29. In addition to medications, use of adaptive aids, such as the wrist splints depicted here, and walking aids can be very helpful with pain and to improve function. These treatments may be applied by physical therapists and occupational therapists as well as physicians. If joints become too damaged, then joint revision or replacement surgery by an orthopedic surgeon may be advised.

PsA: strategizing therapy choice

- Therapy choice based on assessment of disease severity and likelihood of progression
- Current therapy options offer promise of significant control of disease symptoms and signs, as well as risk of disease progression
- Improvement of quality of life and function are key goals of therapy
- Safety and tolerability have improved with emerging therapies, but appropriate surveillance and caution must be maintained
- Patient choice regarding method of administration: oral, subcutaneous, or intravenous

FIGURE 7.30. The goals of therapy of PsA are diminished pain, improvement of function and quality of life, and inhibition of disease progression. Physicians' and patients' choice of therapy must be based on assessment of disease severity and likelihood of progression as well as elements of convenience and preference. Safety and tolerability have improved with the emergence of the new biologic therapies, but appropriate surveillance and caution must be maintained.

References

1. Gladman DD, Farewell VT, Nadeau C. **Clinical indicators of progression in psoriatic arthritis: multivariate relative risk model.** *J Rheumatol* 1995; **22**:675–679.

2. Clegg DO, Reda DJ, Mejias E *et al.* **Comparison of sulfasalazine and placebo in the treatment of psoriatic arthritis. A Department of Veterans Affairs Cooperative Study.** *Arthritis Rheum* 1996; **39**:2013–2020.

3. Mease PJ, Goffe BS, Metz J *et al.* **Etanercept in the treatment of psoriatic arthritis and psoriasis: a randomized trial.** *Lancet* 2000; **356**:385–390.

4. Gladman DD, Helliwell P, Mease PJ *et al.* **Assessment of patients with psoriatic arthritis: a review of currently available measures.** *Arthritis Rheum* 2004; **50**:24–35.

5. Willkens RF, Williams HJ, Ward JR *et al.* **Randomized, double-blind, placebo controlled trial of low-dose pulse methotrexate in psoriatic arthritis.** *Arthritis Rheum* 1984; **27**:376–381.

6. Salvarani C, Macchioni P, Olivieri I *et al.* **A comparison of cyclosporine, sulfasalazine, and symptomatic therapy in the treatment of psoriatic arthritis.** *J Rheumatol* 2001; **28**:2274–2282.

7. Palit J, Hill J, Capell HA *et al.* **A multicentre double-blind comparison of auranofin, intramuscular gold thiomalate and placebo in patients with psoriatic arthritis.** *Br J Rheumatol* 1990; **29**:280–283.

8. Jones G, Crotty M, Brooks P. *Interventions for Treating Psoriatic Arthritis (Cochrane Review).* Oxford: The Cochrane Library; 2001.

9. Kaltwasser JP, Nash P, Gladman D *et al.* **Efficacy and safety of leflunomide in the treatment of psoriatic arthritis and psoriasis: a multimodal, double-blind, randomized, placebo-controlled clinical trial.** *Arthritis Rheum* 2004; **50**:1939–1950.

10. Smith JB, Haynes MK. **Rheumatoid arthritis – a molecular understanding.** *Ann Intern Med* 2002; **136**:908–922.

11. Choy EH, Panayi GS. **Cytokine pathways and joint inflammation in rheumatoid arthritis.** *N Engl J Med* 2001; **344**:907–916.

12. Mease P, Kivitz A, Burch F *et al.* **Etanercept treatment of psoriatic arthritis: safety, efficacy, and effect on disease progression.** *Arth Rheum* 2004; **50**:2264–2272.

13. Antoni C, Krueger GG, de Vlam K *et al.* **Infliximab improves signs and symptoms of psoriatic arthritis: results of the IMPACT 2 trial.** *Ann Rheum Dis* 2005; **64**:1150–1157.

14. Mease PJ, Gladman DD, Ritchlin C *et al.* **Adalimumab therapy in patients with psoriatic arthritis: 24-week results of a phase III study.** *Arthritis Rheum* 2004; **50**:4097 (Abstract).

15. Mease PJ, Gladman DD, Ritchlin C *et al.* **Adalimumab for the treatment of patients with moderately to severely active psoriatic arthritis. Results of a double-blind, randomized, placebo-controlled trial.** *Arthritis Rheum* 2005; **52**:3279–3289.

16. Mease P, Ganguly R, Wanke L *et al.* **How much improvement in pain is considered important by patients with active psoriatic arthritis?** *Ann Rheum Dis* 2004; **63**(Suppl 1):391.

17. Mease PJ, Gladman DD, Ritchlin CT *et al.* **Adalimumab is effective against skin and joint disease in psoriatic arthritis patients: 48-week results of ADEPT.** *Rheumatology* 2006; **45**(Suppl1): 68 (Abstract 129).

18. Nickoloff BJ. **The immunologic and genetic basis of psoriasis.** *Arch Dermatol* 1999; **135**:1104–1110.

19. Mease PJ, Gladman DD, Keystone E. **Efficacy of alefacept in combination with methotrexate in the treatment of psoriatic arthritis.** *Ann Rheum Dis* 2005; **64**:FRI0224.

8
Treatment of Psoriasis

Gerald G. Krueger and Kristina P. Callis

The treatment of psoriasis has long been a challenge to the dermatologist on several levels. Psoriasis does not respond in any predictable fashion to topical or systemic agents, and to date there are no clinical or laboratory measures to predict response to therapy in an individual. In clinical practice, emphasis on impact of the disease and its treatment on a patient's quality of life and health should guide treatment choices. Severity of disease, including location and body surface area, response to previous therapies, medical history, concomitant medications, treatment goals, convenience of administration, and financial limitations, must all be considered carefully when choosing initial therapy. Because in any given patient severity and impact of disease will fluctuate over time and with different therapies, frequent reassessment of symptoms, treatment satisfaction, and short- and long-term side effects of therapy is a necessary approach.

The armamentarium of therapies for psoriasis of any severity is broad in choice and complexity. Traditionally, topical therapies are usually considered first for mild disease. Systemic therapy, including ultraviolet therapy, oral immunosuppressive agents, and biologic agents, or combinations of the above, are considered when patients have more moderate-to-severe disease, or psoriasis that is unresponsive or inappropriate for topical agents.

Definition of the PASI

To calculate a patient's PASI, the severity of erythema, induration, scale, and area affected is assessed in each of the following four anatomic sites:

Head (H)   Upper extremities (U)   Trunk (T)   Lower extremities (L)

These roughly correspond to 10%, 20%, 30%, and 40% of BSA, respectively, and are weighted in the equation accordingly

Erythema (E), induration (I), and scale (S) are assessed according to a 5-point scale:

0: no symptoms   1: slight   2: moderate   3: marked   4: very marked

A is assigned a numerical value based on the extent of lesions in a given anatomic site:

1 = <10%   4 = 50–<70%

2 = 10–<30%   5 = 70–<90%

3 = 30–<50%   6 = 90–100%

For example, if 25% of the trunk is affected with psoriasis, the area of the trunk score or A_T is '2'

The PASI score is then calculated from the following equation:

$$PASI = 0.1(E_H + I_H + S_H)A_H + 0.2(E_U + I_U + S_U)A_U + 0.3(E_T + I_T + S_T)A_T + 0.4(E_L + I_L + S_L)A_L$$

Example of PASI calculation

	Head/neck	Upper extremities	Trunk	Lower extremities	
Erythema	1	2	3	3	
Induration	2	1	2	3	
Scale	+3	+2	+3	+2	
Sum of E, I, S	6	5	8	8	
Sums multiplied by the area score and by multiplier corresponding to that area	x1 x0.1	x2 x0.2	x3 x0.3	x3 x0.4	
then totaled	0.6	+2.0	+7.2	+9.6	= 19.4

FIGURE 8.1. With the ongoing development of new therapies for the treatment of psoriasis, the assessment of psoriasis improvement has become an important focus of researchers and clinicians. What constitutes meaningful improvement of psoriasis remains an active area of study. A number of tools are available to quantify the degree of erythema, thickness, and scaling of lesions, body surface area (BSA) affected, and improvement of quality of life. In the research setting, the most commonly accepted assessment tool is the Psoriasis Area and Severity Index (PASI) [1]. The PASI was developed and first published after its use in a trial of etretinate. It incorporates the severity of erythema, scale, and thickness of plaques and BSA into a mathematically derived score ranging from 0 to 72. Improvement of PASI from baseline by 75% (PASI 75) has been the benchmark needed to bring many biologic agents to market. In a review by Naldi et al., it was noted that 44 different scoring systems were used in 171 randomized clinical trials of psoriasis therapies between 1997 and 2000; PASI was used in roughly half of these trials [2]. However, PASI has numerous limitations and therefore other scoring systems such as the National Psoriasis Foundation Psoriasis Score [3], the Lattice System Physician's Global Assessment (LS-PGA) [4], and numerous versions of the Physician Global Assessment have been developed and validated in large clinical trials. In addition, tools such as the Dermatology Life Quality Index (DLQI) (see Figure 8.2) [5] and psoriasis-specific indices, such as the Psoriasis Disability Index [6] and the Psoriasis Quality of Life Questionnaire 12 [7,8], have been employed to correlate physician-driven scoring systems with quality of life relative to their psoriasis.

Dermatology Life Quality Index

Over the last week, how...	Very much	A lot	A little	Not at all	
1. ...itchy, sore, painful, or stinging has your skin been?	3	2	1	0	
2. ...embarrassed or self-conscious have you been because of your skin?	3	2	1	0	

Over the last week, how...	Very much	A lot	A little	Not at all	Not relevant
3. ...much has your skin interfered with you going shopping or looking after your home or garden?	3	2	1	0	
4. ...much has your skin influenced the clothes you wear?	3	2	1	0	
5. ...much has your skin affected any social or leisure activities?	3	2	1	0	
6. ...much has your skin made it difficult for you to do any sport	3	2	1	0	

Over the last week, has...	Yes	No			Not relevant
7a. ...your skin prevented you from working or studying?	3	0			

If 7a is 'No'...	A lot	A little	Not at all	
7b. ...has your skin been a problem at work or studying?	2	1	0	

Over the last week, how...	Very much	A lot	A little	Not at all	Not relevant
8. ...much has your skin created problems with your partner or any of your close friends or relatives?	3	2	1	0	
9. ...much has your skin caused any sexual difficulties?	3	2	1	0	
10. ...much of a problem has the treatment for your skin been, for example by making your home messy or by taking up time?	3	2	1	0	

FIGURE 8.2.

Topical therapies for psoriasis

Therapeutic class	Examples of vehicles/compounds	Common uses	Cutaneous adverse events	Systemic adverse events
Corticosteroids:				
Class I	**Creams, ointments** Clobetasol propionate 0.05%; halobetasol propionate 0.05%; betamethasone dipropionate 0.05%; diflorasone diacetate 0.05%	Trunk and extremities: twice daily application of cream or ointment as initial treatment, then maintenance (weekends only or every other week in combination with vitamin D analog)	Atrophy, striae, telangiectasia, irritation, tachyphylaxis, rebound, acneiform eruptions, rosacea, folliculitis, contact dermatitis, purpura/ecchymoses, hypopigmentation infection (bacterial, fungal)	Systemic absorption with adrenal suppression, Cushing's syndrome, glaucoma
	Solutions/foams Clobetasol propionate 0.05%	Scalp application (once to twice daily)		
	Occlusive tape Flurandrenolide	Localized, lichenified plaques		
Class IV	Betamethasone valerate foam and lotion	Scalp application (once to twice daily)		

FIGURE 8.3.

(Continued)

Therapeutic class	Examples of vehicles/compounds	Common uses	Cutaneous adverse events	Systemic adverse events
Class V–VI	Hydrocortisone butyrate 0.1%, desonide 0.05%	Face, axilla, groin, genitals, body folds (once to twice daily)		
Vitamin D analogs	Calcipotriene 0.0025% and 0.005% ointment cream and solution, calcipotriol	Trunk and extremities: twice daily in combination with corticosteroids or tazarotene Face, axillae, groin, body folds: once to twice daily Scalp: solution once to twice daily	Irritation (burning, erythema), photosensitivity	Hypervitaminosis D and hypercalcemia
Vitamin A analogs	Tazarotene 0.1% and 0.05% gel and cream		Irritation (itching, burning, erythema), thinning of skin, photosensitivity	Teratogenicity
Immunomodulators	Tacrolimus 0.1% and 0.03% ointment, pimecrolimus 5% cream	Face, axillae, groin, genitals, body folds: once to twice daily	Irritation (burning, itching, erythema)	Systemic absorption leading to potential immunosuppression, renal or hepatotoxicity, rare reports of lymphoma in atopic population
Other agents	Anthralin		Irritation, staining of skin and clothing	
	Coal Tar		Irritation, staining, undesirable odor	
	Salicylic acid	Shampoos, in combination with emollients, and with corticosteroids	Irritation	Potential salicylate toxicity
	Emollients	Liberal use for symptomatic relief of dryness, scaling, pruritus	Irritation, contact dermatitis	

FIGURE 8.3. **Continued** Topical therapies for psoriasis are the most widely used agents for psoriasis given their ease of use, low risk, and familiarity to the physician. Although topical agents are typically prescribed as first-line therapy when BSA is <10–20%, they are not always effective nor acceptable for patients with this amount of disease. Application to a large area is time-consuming, costly, and increases risk of adverse effects. The most commonly used topical agents and their adverse effects are outlined in this figure. Suprapotent corticosteroids are the mainstay of topical therapies, having the most potential for clearance or near clearance of lesions when used as single agents or in combination with other agents [9]. However, adverse effects such as atrophy, striae, and lack of compliance limit their quantity, duration, and location of use. The vitamin D analog calcipotriene, is the single most prescribed agent for psoriasis in the USA, but is limited in efficacy when used as a single agent [10]. Calcipotriene is, therefore, best used in combination with corticosteroids [11–13], ultraviolet (UV) light [14], or systemic therapies such as acitretin [15] and cyclosporine [16,17]. Tazarotene, a vitamin A analog, is effective for psoriasis [18,19], but local irritation limits its use as monotherapy. Tazarotene can also be used as a short contact program [20] in combination with topical corticosteroids [21,22] and UV therapy [23–25]. Anthralin, coal tar, and salicylic acid are still used as adjunctive therapies but rarely as single agents.

Overview of phototherapy for psoriasis

Modality	Administration	Advantages	Disadvantages
Broadband UVB (BBUVB)	3–5 treatments / week starting at 50–100% of the MED or dose appropriate for skin type	Few systemic side effects Long-term safety relative to photoaging, skin cancer Better safety profile in pregnancy and lactation	Shorter remission time compared to NBUVB or PUVA
Narrow-band UVB (NBUVB)	2–3 treatments/week using MED or NBUVB protocols [25]	Few systemic side effects Narrow band of light decreases risk of burning May have less risk of photoaging and skin cancer Better safety profile in pregnancy and lactation	Requires longer time per light treatment to achieve minimal erythema (more standing time)
Psoralen (oral) + UVA (PUVA)	2–3 treatments/week Methoxsalen 0.4 mg/kg 1–15 hours before exposure UVA starting doses determined using minimum phototoxic dose (MPD)	Most efficacious for chronic or recalcitrant psoriasis, particularly thicker plaques Less frequent treatments in clearance and maintenance phase than BBUVB Longest remission (4–6 months) vs. BBUVB or NBUVB	Numerous short-term systemic side effects (most commonly GI and CNS disturbance) and cutaneous side effects (phototoxicity, pruritus, erythema, photoeruptions, Koebner phenomenon, herpes simplex) Must avoid natural UV exposure of eyes and skin for 8–12 hours post ingestion of psoralen Long-term side effects including cataracts, increased risk of photoaging, freckling, lentigenes, keratoses, telangectasia Long-term increased risk of non-melanoma and melanoma skin cancer, especially type I and II skin

FIGURE 8.4.

(Continued)

Modality	Administration	Advantages	Disadvantages
Topical psoralen (bath, soak, cream) + UVA	2–3 treatments/week Bathing/soaking in water with methoxsalen to water, then immediate UVA exposure based on MPD Cream: application of cream with subsequent UVA exposure	Reduced systemic and cutaneous symptoms compared to PUVA May be as or more efficacious than PUVA Provides more focal therapy for limited or localized disease	Inconvenience and mess of bathing or application of cream Phototoxicity, erythema, pain, pruritus still common Sun avoidance still required Limited data on carcinogenesis
Excimer laser	Twice-weekly treatments of 308-nm xenon chloride laser for 6–10 treatments	Good for patients with localized or limited disease, unresponsive to topical disease, or who are non-compliant with topicals Few treatments required	Can only treat limited BSA Side effects include erythema, blistering, hyperpigmentation, erosion Long-term studies not yet available

FIGURE 8.4. **Continued** UV light has long been recognized as effective therapy for psoriasis. Office-based UV, in the form of broadband UVB, narrowband UVB, and UVA combined with systemic or topical psoralen (PUVA) are highly efficacious modalities for psoriasis. The administration and selection of UV therapy is dependent on many factors summarized in this figure. UV light is often combined with topical agents, particularly when scalp or body folds are involved. UV is often combined with topical and systemic agents when UV has not met expectations as a single agent. UV is absolutely contraindicated in patients with photosensitive disease such as lupus, and relatively contraindicated in patients taking photosensitizing medications. Ultimate success of the selected treatment depends on the technical expertise of the physician and staff, the physical and financial accessibility of the light boxes, compliance of the patient, and general responsiveness of disease to UV.

UVB is still considered first-line therapy for moderate-to-severe psoriasis, particularly if the disease is generalized and/or unresponsive to topical agents. UVB is considered relatively safer than PUVA and systemic agents such as methotrexate and cyclosporine, particularly in certain populations such as females that are pregnant or lactating, or individuals with liver or renal disease. Dosing is based on Fitzpatrick skin type or minimal erythema dose (MED), and is usually administered three to five times per week. Narrow-band UVB (311–313 nm) is increasingly being used in place of broadband UVB. It has been shown to be more efficacious than broadband UVB, and can be administered less frequently (two to three times per week) [26].

PUVA, or the use of the photosensitizing oral methoxsalen with subsequent exposure to UVA (320–400 nm), is a highly effective therapy for psoriasis. Its exact mechanism of action in psoriasis is unknown, but the suspected role is formation of pyrimidine dimers and subsequent cross-linkage of DNA and death of inflammatory cells. Since it penetrates more deeply it is often recommended for patients with chronic, thicker plaque disease. It is more effective than broadband UVB, requires less frequency of visits, and can better treat nail disease or palmar/plantar disease. Topical psoralen administered as bath, soak, or cream, used more widely in Europe, has the advantages of treating localized disease without increased risk of gastrointestinal (GI) or ophthalmologic side effects and skin cancer.

The excimer laser is a xenon-chloride laser that produces UV light at the 308-nm wavelength, providing a localized form of UV near the peak of the psoriasis improvement spectrum. The nickel-sized spot size limits therapy to only a few plaques per session, thereby restricting its use to patients with localized disease. In one series 72% (66/92) of subjects achieved 75% clearing with an average of 6.2 treatments [27]. CNS, central nervous system.

Overview of systemic agents for psoriasis

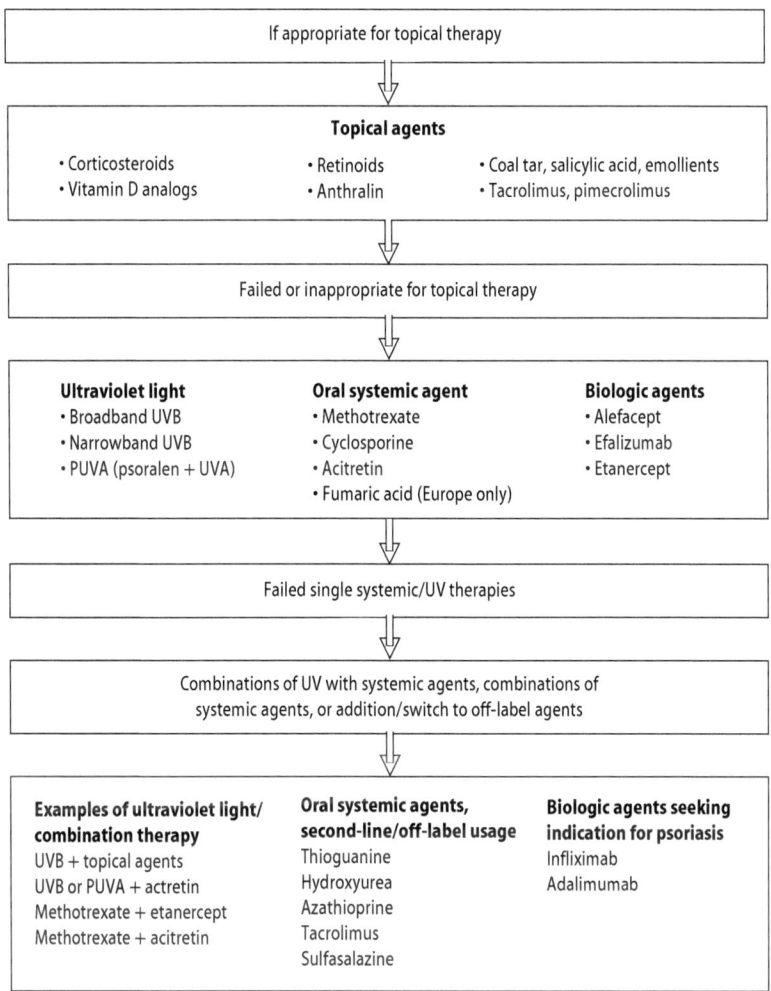

FIGURE 8.5. Systemic therapies for psoriasis are often chosen for patients with moderate-to-severe psoriasis who have failed, or are not good candidates for, UV therapy. The most commonly used oral systemic agents are methotrexate, cyclosporine, and acitretin.

Methotrexate, a dihydrofolate reductase inhibitor, has been used for the treatment of psoriasis since the late 1950s [28]. It has been considered highly effective therapy for psoriasis; however, no rigorous clinical trials were ever conducted prior to its USA Food and Drug Administration approval. A recent comparative trial of cyclosporine versus methotrexate suggested comparable efficacy between the two agents [29]. Methotrexate is usually administered in weekly or twice weekly regimens, at doses ranging from 5 mg to 30 mg/week. Toxicity, including nausea, mouth sores, asthenia, bone marrow toxicity, hepatotoxicity, and rare pneumonitis, limit its short- and long-term use. It is also teratogenic and known to cause miscarriages.

Cyclosporine is a calcineurin inhibitor that works by inhibiting interleukin (IL)-2 production, thereby preventing activation and proliferation of T-cells [30]. Cyclosporine is a highly effective therapy for psoriasis [31]. Because of its short- and long-term toxicities, it is recommended for short-term use, usually in the setting of a sudden, severe, or recalcitrant flare of psoriasis. It is usually administered in doses of 3–5 mg/kg. Side effects include neuropathy, GI disturbance, nephrotoxicity, hypertension, hyperlipidemia, hypomagnesemia, hyperkalemia, susceptibility to infection, and long-term risk of lymphoproliferative disorders and cutaneous malignancy.

Acitretin is a systemic oral retinoid that replaced its predecessor, etretinate, in 1997. It is usually administered in doses of 25–50 mg/day. It is highly effective for pustular psoriasis. As a single agent for plaque psoriasis its efficacy is limited unless administered at high doses; therefore, it is often used in conjunction with phototherapy [32,33]. Side effects tend to be more problematic at higher doses, particularly mucocutaneous symptoms such as dry lips and skin, cheilitis, 'sticky skin', and hair loss. Because it is teratogenic, it is absolutely contraindicated in females of childbearing potential. Monitoring must be done for hyperlipidemia, particularly hypertriglyceridemia, and abnormal liver function tests. Osteoporosis, ligamentous calcification skeletal problems, and rare cases of pseudotumor cerebri are associated with acitretin use.

Other systemic therapies, such as thioguanine, sulfasalazine, hydroxyurea, azathioprine, tacrolimus, and mycophenolate mofetil, have been used to treat psoriasis off-label but no large clinical trials support their use.

Biologic agents currently available or in late-phase trials for psoriasis

Agent	Approval status	Administration	Efficacy	Safety and monitoring
Alefacept	USA: approved for moderate-to-severe psoriasis	15 mg IM weekly in office for 12 weeks, followed by 12-week break then second 12-week course	PASI 75: 33% at week 14, 43% after second course	Flu-like symptoms (chills); monitor CD4$^+$ lymphocyte counts weekly, hold dosing for CD4 count <250 cells/μl
Efalizumab	USA: approved for moderate-to-severe plaque psoriasis	0.7 mg/kg loading dose, then weekly 1 mg/kg subcutaneous injections by patient	PASI 75: 28% at week 12, 44% at week 24	Flu-like symptoms with initial doses Monitor platelet counts Potential for rebound if stopped abruptly
Etanercept	USA: approved for juvenile and adult rheumatoid arthritis (RA), psoriatic arthritis (PsA), ankylosing spondylitis, moderate-to-severe psoriasis	25 mg and 50 mg subcutaneous injection twice weekly by patient	PASI 75: for 25 mg, 32–34% at week 12, 44–45% at week 24; for 50 mg, 46–49% at week 12, 59% at week 24 [37,38], 51% at week 96 [39]	Injection site reactions (etanercept and adalimumab) Infusion reactions including anaphylaxis (infliximab) monitoring for demyelinating disorders, lupus, hematologic disorders Tuberculosis testing including PPD and/or chest radiography
Infliximab	USA: RA, Crohn's, PsA; in phase III trials for psoriasis and ankylosing spondylitis	5 mg/kg IV infusion at weeks 0, 2, and 6 followed by every 8 weeks for maintenance	PASI 75: 80% at week 10, 82% at week 24, 61% at week 50 [40]	Bacterial and mycobacterial infections (all anti-TNF-α agents) Neutralizing antibodies (infliximab)
Adalimumab	USA: RA; in phase III trials for psoriasis and PsA	40 mg every other week subcutaneous injection by patient	PASI 75: 53% at week 12, 64% at week 24, 58% at week 60 [41]	

FIGURE 8.6. Since psoriasis is a chronic, often lifetime disease, the need for therapy that can be used chronically has driven the development of numerous targeted therapies. Although the pathogenesis of psoriasis is complex and not fully understood, therapeutic strategies based on the major events that lead to psoriasis have been developed and have led to the development of the biologic agents summarized in this figure [34–36]. Essentially, for psoriasis to develop, several processes must occur: 1) T-cells must migrate to the skin via adhesion to skin-specific receptors on endothelium; 2) T-cells must be activated by specific chemokines and receptor interactions; 3) genetically predisposed skin responds to cytokines, for example, tumor necrosis factor (TNF)-α, generated by the immune cell interaction in a manner that leads to the histopathology of a psoriatic lesion.

Two of the biologic agents effective in psoriasis interfere with the upstream T-cell mechanisms; efalizumab targets both the migration of T-cells and interference with the costimulatory response, while alefacept antagonizes the costimulatory response to prevent activation of memory T-cells as well as reducing the number of activated T-cells via apoptotic mechanisms through the perforin-granzyme system. Alternatively, the anti-TNF-α agents interrupt the downstream immune activation by neutralizing the pro-inflammatory cytokine TNF-α. IM, intramuscular; IV, intravenous; PPD, purified protein derivative.

Alefacept, a fully humanized fusion protein

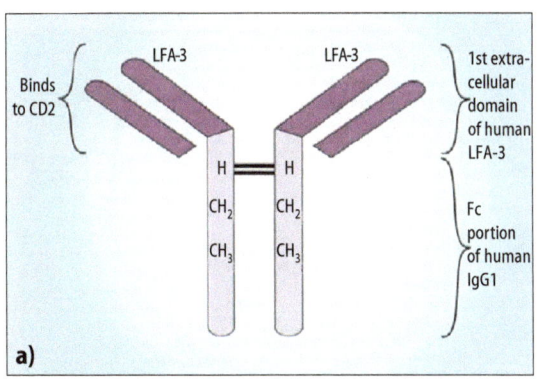

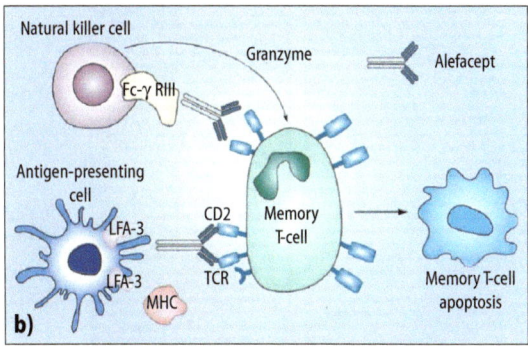

FIGURE 8.7. Alefacept (Amevive®; Biogen, Inc., Cambridge, MA, USA) was the first biologic agent approved in the USA for treatment of plaque-type psoriasis. It is a fully humanized fusion protein consisting of the extracellular domain of lymphocyte function-associated antigen-3 (LFA-3) fused to the hinge, the CH2 domain, and the CH3 domain of immunoglobulin (Ig)G1 **(a)** [42]. It is believed to have a dual mechanism of action in psoriasis **(b)**. The LFA-3 portion of alefacept binds to CD2 receptors on T-cells, inter-fering with the LFA-3–CD2 co-stimulatory response. The IgG1 portion binds to the Fc-γ receptor (Fc-γR) on natural killer cells facilitating granzyme-mediated apoptosis of activated memory T-cells [43,44]. The prolonged remission seen in some psoriasis patients has been attributed to targeted apoptosis of the memory T-cell population in which CD2 is upregulated [45,46]. MHC, major histocompatibility complex; TCR, T-cell receptor.

PASI response and efficacy of alefacept in two phase III studies

a)

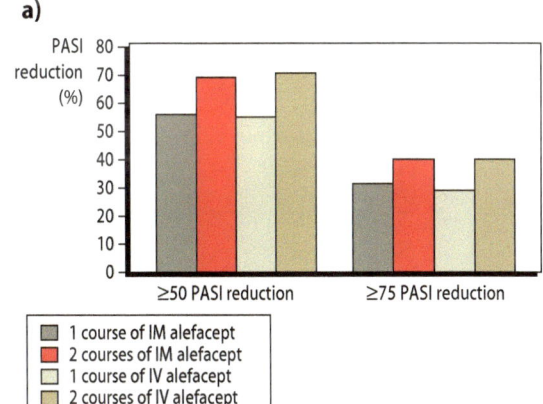

b)

Dose	Efficacy outcome (& of patients)*		
	≥50 reduction in PASI (%)	≥75 reduction in PASI (%)	PGA of 'clear' of 'almost clear' (%)
Alefacept 7.5 mg IV (n=367)	56†	28†	23†
Placebo (n=186)	24	8	6
Alefacept 15 mg IM (n=166)	57†	33†	24†
Placebo (n=168)	35	13	8

FIGURE 8.8. *Assessed throughout the study period. †$p < 0.01$. The efficacy, safety, and durability of response to alefacept has been demonstrated in the clinical trials leading to its approval for use in plaque-type psoriasis. A phase II, randomized, double-blind, multicenter dose-ranging trial of 229 patients with plaque-type psoriasis revealed that the percentage of patients reaching at least 50% reduction from baseline PASI (PASI 50) were 36%, 60%, and 56% for patients receiving alefacept IV 0.025, 0.075, and 0.150 mg/kg weekly for 12 weeks, respectively, compared with 25% for the placebo group [47]. The approval of alefacept in the USA was based on the two subsequent phase III studies. **(a)** Shows the PASI 50 and 75 response after one or two courses of alefacept, and **(b)** shows the efficacy of one 12-week course of IV and IM alefacept [47,48]. In the IV study, 553 patients were randomized to receive alefacept 7.5 mg or placebo in two 12-week courses [48], and in the IM study, 507 patients received a single 12-week course of alefacept (10 mg or 15 mg weekly) or placebo. PASI 75 for one or two courses at any time point of alefacept IM is 33% and 43%, and of alefacept IV is 28% and 56%, respectively. Alefacept also has the potential for a longer remission than most other systemic agents [49]. There are few short- or long-term effects. However, drawbacks include the need for IM injection, cost, and weekly monitoring for drop in CD4+ T-cell counts. PGA, Physician's Global Assessment. Modified from [50].

PASI 75 response to etanercept in a phase II trial

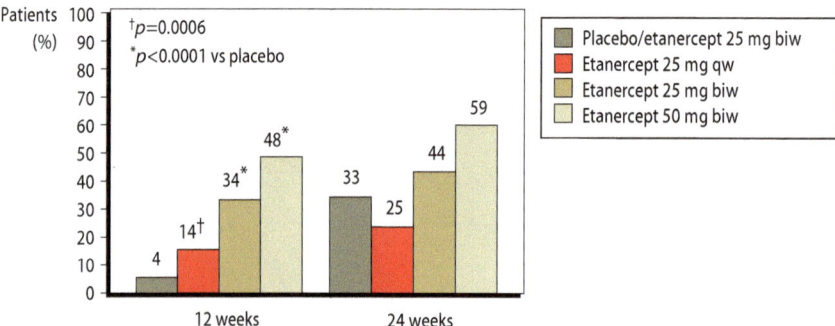

FIGURE 8.9. Etanercept (Enbrel®; Amgen Inc., Thousand Oaks, CA, USA) is a fully humanized dimeric fusion protein consisting of the 75-kD TNF receptor linked to the Fc portion of human IgG1. It is believed to work by neutralizing TNF-α, which plays a significant role in the pathogenesis of psoriasis [51]. In the pivotal PsA trial, 26% of patients who had at least 3% BSA affected achieved an improvement in PASI 75. In the pivotal phase II trial, 30% of treated subjects versus 2% receiving placebo reached PASI 75 at 12 weeks, and 56% (vs 5% of the placebo group) reached PASI 75 at 24 weeks [52]. Data from the phase III trial of etanercept 25 mg weekly, 25 mg twice weekly, and 50 mg twice weekly, versus placebo is presented in this figure. At week 24, the PASI 75 was reached by 25% of the low-dose group, 44% of the medium-dose group, and 59% of the high-dose group [37]. This drug is administered subcutaneously at 25–50 mg twice weekly, and ongoing post-marketing studies are evaluating maintenance doses. The most common shortterm side effects are injection site reactions, upper respiratory infection, and headache. biw, twice weekly; qw, weekly. Modified with permission from [37].

Percentage of patients achieving PASI 75 or PASI 50 in efalizumab-treated (1 mg/kg/wk) and placebo groups

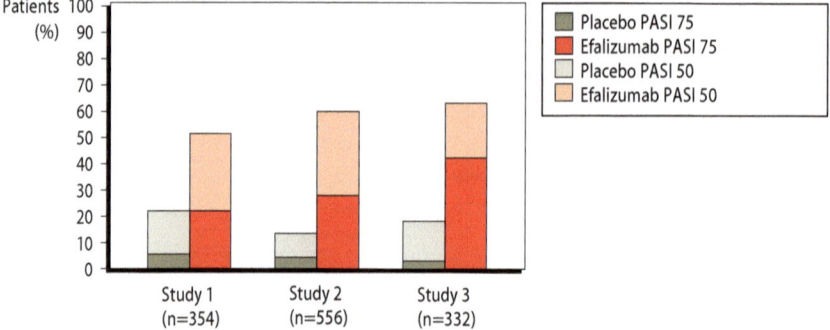

FIGURE 8.10. Efalizumab (Raptiva®; Genentech, Inc., South San Francisco, CA, USA) is a humanized IgG1 monoclonal antibody against CD11a, the α-subunit of LFA-1 [53]. LFA-1 and intercellular adhesion molecule 1 (ICAM-1) are costimulatory molecules expressed on T-cells and antigen-presenting cells, respectively, that facilitate multiple T-cell-mediated events. It is felt to work by inhibiting the ICAM-1–LFA-1 interaction that facilitates extravasation of T-lymphocytes into the skin as well as inhibiting the co-stimulatory response that is important to the pathogenesis of psoriasis. Efalizumab is administered as a subcutaneous weekly injection. The figure shows the percentage of patients achieving a 50% or 75% improvement in PASI in clinical trials [54–56]. PASI 75 was achieved in 27% of patients in 3 months, and 44% of patients at 6 months in the extended trial [56,57]. Its most common side effects include flu-like symptoms with the first doses and rare cases of thrombocytopenia, and rebound of psoriasis following withdrawal of the drug in individuals who have not had a good response has occasionally been observed. Reproduced with permission from [58].

Adalimumab efficacy at weeks 12, 24 and 60

PASI 75 response

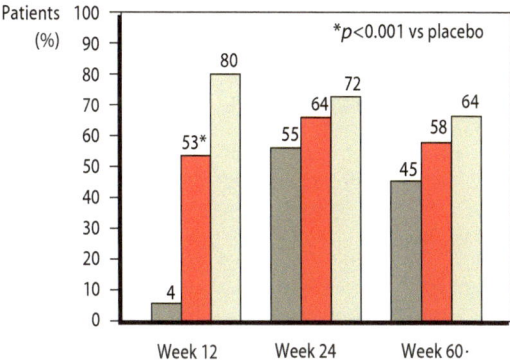

PGA-'clear/almost clear'

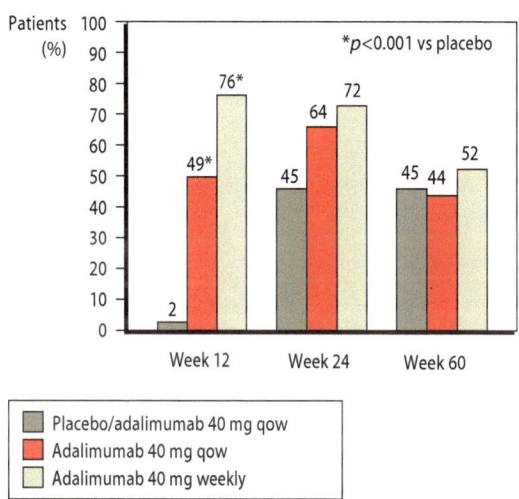

Placebo/adalimumab 40 mg qow
Adalimumab 40 mg qow
Adalimumab 40 mg weekly

FIGURE 8.11. Adalimumab (Humira®; Abbott Laboratories, North Chicago, IL, USA) is a fully monoclonal IgG1 antibody that targets TNF-α. It is currently approved in the USA, Europe, and elsewhere for the treatment of RA and is under investigation for psoriasis, PsA, and other diseases. In a 12-week, double-blind, placebo-controlled, phase II trial, 148 patients were randomized to receive 80 mg adalimumab at week 0 followed by 40 mg adalimumab every other week (qow); 80 mg adalimumab at weeks 0 and 1, followed by 40 mg weekly; or placebo [41,59]. At week 12, as part of the 48-week extension study, the placebo group received 80 mg adalimumab, then 40 mg qow, and the other two groups continued their same weekly dosing regimen. At week 12, an improvement in PASI 75 or better was achieved in 53% of patients receiving 40 mg qow, 80% of patients receiving 40 mg weekly, and only 4% receiving placebo [41]. At week 24, a PASI 75 or better was achieved in 64% of patients getting low dose, and 72% of patients getting high dose. At week 24, in patients without PsA, 64% of patients given low dose and 72% of patients given high dose were deemed clear/almost clear. A phase III study of the low-dose regimen is underway.

Randomized placebo-controlled trials with infliximab

Study	Regimen	% of patients reaching PASI 75 at primary endpoint	Extension studies or follow-up
IIS phase II (moderate-to-severe plaque psoriasis >5% BSA) [59]	Infliximab 5 mg/kg (n=11), infliximab 10 mg/kg (n=11), placebo (n=11), IV infusions at weeks 0, 2, and 6	81.8% (5 mg/kg), 72.7% (10 mg/kg), 18.2% (placebo) at week 10	Week 10–26 open-label phase: 29 patients re-randomized to 5 mg/kg or 10 mg/kg infusions at week 10, 12, and 16; 5 mg/kg: 33% maintained PASI 75; 10 mg/kg: 67% maintained PASI 75; endpoint at week 26 [58]
IMPACT (Infliximab Multinational Psoriatic Arthritis Controlled Trial; 39 patients with PASI >2.5) [55]	Infliximab 5 mg/kg (n=22), placebo (n=17), IV infusions at weeks 0, 2, 6, and 14; extension study with infusions at weeks 22, 30, 38, and 46; crossover placebo group infusions at weeks 16, 18, 22, 30, 38, and 46	68% (5 mg/kg) vs 0% of placebo at week 16	At week 50, infliximab/infliximab group (n=22) PASI 75 sustained in 59%; placebo/infliximab group (n=16) 50% reached PASI 75
IMPACT 2 (subjects with BSA >3%) [56]	Infliximab 5 mg/kg (n=83), placebo (n=87)	63.9% (5 mg/kg) vs. 2% of placebo at week 14	
SPIRIT (Study of Psoriasis with Infliximab Induction Therapy) [57]	Infliximab 3 mg/kg (n=99), infliximab 5 mg/kg (n=99), placebo (n=51) at 0, 2, and 6 weeks	71.7% (3 mg/kg), 87.9% (5 mg/kg), 5.9% (placebo) at week 10	14% of 3-mg/kg group and 30% of 5-mg/kg group maintained PASI 75 at week 26

FIGURE 8.12. Infliximab (Remicade®; Malvern, PA, USA) is a monoclonal antibody comprised of mouse variable region and a human IgG1/α-constant region, with high specificity, affinity, and avidity for TNF. It is currently approved in the USA for the treatment of RA, Crohn's disease, and PsA, and is in phase III studies for plaque-type psoriasis and ankylosing spondylitis. Randomized controlled studies of infliximab for psoriasis are presented in this figure. All studies have shown infliximab to be highly efficacious for moderate-to-severe plaque psoriasis [60–64]. Infliximab is administered at doses of 3, 5, and 10 mg/kg over 2–3 hours via IV infusion. Antibodies to infliximab have been known to develop after induction therapy. The titers of antibodies are generally low, but have been shown to limit efficacy of treatment and may increase incidence of adverse events [65]. Regular maintenance dosing with infliximab, higher doses of infliximab, and treatment with concomitant immunosuppressives, such as methotrexate, have been shown to reduce development of antiinfliximab antibodies [66,67]. IIS, investigator initiated study.

References

1. Fredriksson T, Pettersson U. **Severe psoriasis – oral therapy with a new retinoid.** *Dermatologica* 1978; 157:238–244.
2. Naldi L, Svensson A, Diepgen T *et al.* **European Dermato-Epidemiology Network. Randomized clinical trials for psoriasis 1977–2000 the EDEN survey.** *J Invest Dermatol* 2003; 120:738–741.
3. Krueger GG. **New method being developed for assessing psoriasis.** *National Psoriasis Foundation Forum* 1999; 5:4–5.
4. Langley RG, Ellis CN. **Evaluating psoriasis with Psoriasis Area and Severity Index, Psoriasis Global Assessment, and Lattice System Physician's Global Assessment.** *J Am Acad Dermatol* 2004; 51:563–569.
5. Finlay AY, Khan GK. **Dermatology Life Quality Index (DLQI) – a simple practical measure for routine clinical use.** *Clin Exp Dermatol* 1994; 19:210–216.
6. Finlay AY, Kelly SE. **Psoriasis – an index of disability.** *Clin Exp Dermatol* 1987; 12:8–11.
7. Koo J, Menter A, Lebwohl M *et al.* **The relationship between quality of life and disease severity: results from a large cohort of mild, moderate, and severe psoriasis patients.** *Br J Dermatol* 2002; 147:1078.
8. Koo J, Kozma CM, Menter A *et al.* **Development of a disease specific quality of life questionnaire – the 12-item Psoriasis Quality of Life Questionnaire**

(PQOL-12). Presented at: *61st Annual Meeting of the American Academy of Dermatology.* San Francisco, CA. March 21–26, 2003.

9. Katz HI, Hien NT, Prawer SE *et al.* **Superpotent topical steroid treatment of psoriasis vulgaris – clinical efficacy and adrenal function.** *J Am Acad Dermatol* 1987; 16:804–811.

10. Bruce S, Epinette WW, Funicella T *et al.* **Comparative study of calcipotriene (MC 903) ointment and fluocinonide ointment in the treatment of psoriasis.** *J Am Acad Dermatol* 1994; 31(5, Pt 1):755–759.

11. Lebwohl M, Siskin SB, Epinette W *et al.* **A multicenter trial of calcipotriene ointment and halobetasol ointment compared with either agent alone for the treatment of psoriasis.** *J Am Acad Dermatol* 1996; 35(2, Pt 1):268–269.

12. Lebwohl M, Yoles A, Lombardi K *et al.* **Calcipotriene ointment and halobetasol ointment in the long-term treatment of psoriasis: effects on the duration of improvement.** *J Am Acad Dermatol* 1998; 39:447–450.

13. Singh S, Reddy DC, Pandey SS. **Topical therapy for psoriasis with the use of augmented betamethasone and calcipotriene on alternate weeks.** *J Am Acad Dermatol* 2000; 43(1, Pt 1):61–65.

14. Ramsay CA, Schwartz BE, Lowson D *et al.* **Calcipotriol cream combined with twice weekly broad-band UVB phototherapy: a safe, effective and UVB-sparing antipsoriatric combination treatment. The Canadian Calcipotriol and UVB Study Group.** *Dermatology* 2000; 200:17–24.

15. van de Kerkhof PC, Cambazard F, Hutchinson PE *et al.* **The effect of addition of calcipotriol ointment (50 micrograms/g) to acitretin therapy in psoriasis.** *Br J Dermatol* 1998; 138:84–89.

16. Grossman RM, Thivolet J, Claudy A *et al.* **A novel therapeutic approach to psoriasis with combination calcipotriol ointment and very low-dose cyclosporine: results of a multicenter placebo-controlled study.** *J Am Acad Dermatol* 1994; 31:68–74.

17. Kokelj F, Torsello P, Plozzer C. **Calcipotriol improves the efficacy of cyclosporine in the treatment of psoriasis vulgaris.** *J Eur Acad Dermatol Venereol* 1998; 10:143–146.

18. Duvic M, Asano AT, Hager C *et al.* **The pathogenesis of psoriasis and the mechanism of action of tazarotene.** *J Am Acad Dermatol* 1998; 39(4, Pt 2): S129–S133.

19. Krueger GG, Drake LA, Elias PM *et al.* **The safety and efficacy of tazarotene gel, a topical acetylenic retinoid, in the treatment of psoriasis.** *Arch Dermatol* 1998; 134:57–60.

20. Persaud A, Bershad S, Lamba S *et al.* **Short contact tazarotene therapy for psoriasis.** Poster presented at: *American Academy of Dermatology.* Nashville, TN, 2000.

21. Koo JY, Martin D. **Investigator-masked comparison of tazarotene gel q.d. plus mometasone furoate cream q.d. vs. mometasone furoate cream b.i.d. in the treatment of plaque psoriasis.** *Int J Dermatol* 2001; 40:210–212.

22. Lebwohl M, Lombardi K, Tan MH. **Duration of improvement in psoriasis after treatment with tazarotene 0.1% gel plus clobetasol propionate 0.05% ointment: comparison of maintenance treatments.** *Int J Dermatol* 2001; 40:64–66.

23. Lowe NJ. **Optimizing therapy: tazarotene in combination with phototherapy.** *Br J Dermatol* 1999; 140(Suppl 54):8–11.

24. Koo JY, Lowe NJ, Lew-Kaya DA *et al.* **Tazarotene plus UVB phototherapy in the treatment of psoriasis.** *J Am Acad Dermatol* 2000; 43(5, Pt 1):821–828.

25. Behrens S, Grundmann-Kollmann M, Schiener R *et al.* **Combination phototherapy of psoriasis with narrow-band UVB irradiation and topical tazarotene gel.** *J Am Acad Dermatol* 2000; 42:493–495.

26. Shelk J, Morgan P. **Narrow-band UVB: a practical approach.** *Dermatol Nurs* 2000; 12:407–411.

27. Feldman SR, Mellen BG, Housman TS *et al.* **Efficacy of the 308-nm excimer laser for treatment of psoriasis: results of a multicenter study.** *J Am Acad Dermatol* 2002; 46:900–906.

28. Gubner R. **Effect of aminopterin on epithelial tissues.** *Arch Dermatol* 1951; 64:699.

29. Heydendael VM, Spuls PI, Opmeer BC *et al.* **Methotrexate versus cyclosporine in moderate-to-severe chronic plaque psoriasis.** *N Engl J Med* 2003; 349:658–665.

30. Granelli-Piperno A, Nolan P, Inaba K *et al.* **The effect of immunosuppressive agents on the induction of nuclear factors that bind to sites on the interleukin 2 promoter.** *J Exp Med* 1990; 172:1869–1872.

31. Ellis CN, Gorsulowsky DC, Hamilton TA *et al.* **Cyclosporine improves psoriasis in a double-blind study.** *JAMA* 1986; 256:3110–3116.

32. Tanew A, Guggenbichler A, Honigsmann H *et al.* **Photochemotherapy for severe psoriasis without or in combination with acitretin: a randomized, double-blind comparison study.** *J Am Acad Dermatol* 1991; 25:682–684.

33. Lowe NJ, Prystowsky JH, Bourget T *et al.* **Acitretin plus UVB therapy for psoriasis. Comparisons with placebo plus UVB and acitretin alone.** *J Am Acad Dermatol* 1991; 24:591–594.

34. Mehlis SL, Gordon KB. **The immunology of psoriasis and biologic immunotherapy.** *J Am Acad Dermatol* 2003; 49:S44–S50.

35. Singri P, West DP, Gordon KB. **Biologic therapy for psoriasis: the new therapeutic frontier.** *Arch Dermatol* 2002; **138**:657–663.

36. Krueger JG. **The immunologic basis for the treatment of psoriasis with new biologic agents.** *J Am Acad Dermatol* 2002; **46**:1–23.

37. Leonardi CL, Powers JL, Metheson RT *et al.* **For the Etanercept Psoriasis Study Group. Etanercept as monotherapy in patients with psoriasis.** *N Engl J Med* 2003; **349**:2014–2022.

38. Papp KA, Tyring S, Lahfa M *et al.* **A global phase III randomized controlled trial of etanercept in psoriasis: safety, efficacy, and effect of dose reduction.** *Br J Dermatol* 2005; **152**:1304–1312.

39. Tyring S, Poulin Y, Langley R *et al.* **A 96-week phase 3 study of safety and efficacy of etanercept 50 mg twice weekly in patients with psoriasis.** Presented at: *64th Annual Meeting of the American Academy of Dermatology;* San Francisco, CA; March 3–7, 2006; Poster P39.

40. Reich K, Nestle FO, Papp K *et al.* **Infliximab induction and maintenance therapy for moderate-to-severe psoriasis: a phase III, multicentre, double-blind trial.** *Lancet* 2005; **366**:1367–1374.

41. Langley R, Leonardi C, Okun M. **Long-term safety and efficacy of adalimumab in psoriasis.** Presented at: *European Academy of Dermatology and Venereology Spring Symposium.* Lapland, Finland; February 9–12, 2006.

42. *Amevive® (Alefacept) Product Information.* Biogen Inc., MA, USA.

43. Majeau GR, Meier W, Jimmo B *et al.* **Mechanism of lymphocyte function-associated molecule 3-Ig fusion proteins inhibition of T-cell responses. Structure/function analysis** *in vitro* **and in human CD2 transgenic mice.** *J Immunol* 1994; **152**:2753–2767.

44. Miller GT, Hochman PS, Meier W *et al.* **Specific interaction of lymphocyte function-associated antigen 3 with CD2 can inhibit T-cell responses.** *J Exp Med* 1993; **178**:211–222.

45. Krueger GG, Papp KA, Stough DB *et al.* **A randomized, double-blind, placebo-controlled phase III study evaluating efficacy and tolerability of 2 courses of alefacept in patients with chronic plaque psoriasis.** *J Am Acad Dermatol* 2002; **47**:821–833.

46. Gordon KB, Langley RG. **Remitive effects of intramuscular alefacept in psoriasis.** *J Drugs Dermatol* 2003; **2**:624–628.

47. Ellis CN, Krueger GG. **Treatment of chronic plaque psoriasis by selective targeting of memory effector T lymphocytes.** *N Engl J Med* 2001; **345**:248–255.

48. Krueger GG, Papp KA, Stough DB *et al.* **A randomized, double-blind, placebo-controlled phase III** study evaluating efficacy and tolerability of 2 courses of alefacept in patients with chronic plaque psoriasis. *J Am Acad Dermatol* 2002; **47**:821–833.

49. Lebwohl M, Christophers E, Langley R *et al.* **An international, randomized, double-blind, placebo-controlled phase 3 trial of intramuscular alefacept in patients with chronic plaque psoriasis.** *Arch Dermatol* 2003; **139**:719–727.

50. Krueger GG. **Current concepts and review of alefacept in the treatment of psoriasis.** *Dermatol Clin* 2004; **22**:407–426, viii.

51. Robert C, Kupper TS. **Inflammatory skin diseases, T cells, and immune surveillance.** *N Engl J Med* 1999; **341**:1817–1828.

52. Gottlieb AB, Matheson RT, Lowe N *et al.* **A randomized trial of etanercept as monotherapy for psoriasis.** *Arch Dermatol* 2003; **139**:1627–1632.

53. Werther WA, Gonzalez TN, O'Connor SJ *et al.* **Humanization of an anti-lymphocyte function-associated antigen (LFA-1) monoclonal antibody and reengineering of the humanized antibody for binding to rhesus LFA-1.** *J Immunol* 1996; **157**:4986–4995.

54. Lebwohl M, Tyring SK, Hamilton TK *et al.* **A novel targeted T-cell modulator, efalizumab, for plaque psoriasis.** *N Engl J Med* 2003; **349**:2004–2013.

55. Gordon KB, Papp KA, Hamilton TK *et al.* **Efalizumab for patients with moderate to severe plaque psoriasis: a randomized controlled trial.** *JAMA* 2003; **290**:3073–3080.

56. Leonardi CL, Papp KA, Gordon KB *et al.* **Extended efalizumab therapy improves chronic plaque psoriasis: results from a randomized phase III trial.** *J Am Acad Dermatol* 2005; **52**(3, Pt 1):425–433.

57. Menter A, Gordon K, Carey W *et al.* **Efficacy and safety observed during 24 weeks of efalizumab therapy in patients with moderate to severe plaque psoriasis.** *Arch Dermatol* 2005; **141**:31–38.

58. Marano CW, Evans R, Guzzo C *et al.* **Immunogenicity of infliximab (Remicade®) and its effect on safety in patients with severe plaque-type psoriasis.** Presented at: *61st Annual Meeting of the American Academy of Dermatology.* San Francisco, CA; March 21–26, 2003.

59. Menter A, Gordon K, Leonardi C *et al.* **Adalimumab efficacy and safety results in patients with moderate to severe chronic plaque psoriasis with and without psoriatic arthritis.** Poster presented at: *American Academy of Dermatology Annual Meeting.* New Orleans, LA; February 18–22, 2005. Poster 2713.

60. Antoni CE, Kavanaugh A, Kirkham B *et al.* **Sustained benefits of infliximab therapy for dermato-**

logic and articular manifestations of psoriatic arthritis: results from the infliximab multinational psoriatic arthritis controlled trial (IMPACT). *Arthritis Rheum* 2005; **52**:1227–1236.

61. Antoni C, Krueger GG, de Vlam K *et al.* **Infliximab improves signs and symptoms of psoriatic arthritis: results of the IMPACT 2 trial.** *Ann Rheum Dis* 2005; **54**:1227–1236.

62. Gottlieb AB, Evans R, Li S *et al.* **Infliximab induction therapy for patients with severe plaque-type psoriasis: a randomized, double-blind, placebo-controlled trial.** *J Am Acad Dermatol* 2004; **51**:534–542.

63. Gottlieb AB, Chaudhari U, Mulcahy *et al.* **Infliximab mono-therapy provides rapid and sustained benefit for plaque-type psoriasis.** *J Am Acad Dermatol* 2003; **48**:829–835.

64. Chaudhari U, Romano P, Mulcahy LD *et al.* **Efficacy and safety of infliximab monotherapy for plaque-type psoriasis: a randomised trial.** *Lancet* 2001; **357**:1842–1847.

65. Wagner CL, Schantz A, Barnathan E *et al.* **Consequences of immunogenicity to the therapeutic monoclonal antibodies ReoPro and Remicade.** *Dev Biol* 2003; **2**:37–53.

66. Maini RN, Breedveld FC, Kalden JR *et al.* **Therapeutic efficacy of multiple intravenous infusions of anti-tumor necrosis factor alpha monoclonal antibody combined with low-dose weekly methotrexate in rheumatoid arthritis.** *Arthritis Rheum* 1998; **41**:1552–1563.

67. Leonardi CL. **Current concepts and review of efalizumab in the treatment of psoriasis.** *Dermatol Clin* 2004; **22**:427–435.

Index